Stellar
Medicine

A Journey Through
the Universe of Women's Health

By Saralyn Mark, M.D.

Brick Tower Press
Habent Sua Fata Libelli

Brick Tower Press
1230 Park Avenue
New York, New York 10128
Tel: 212-427-7139 • Fax: 212-860-8852
bricktower@aol.com • www.BrickTowerPress.com

Library of Congress Cataloging-in-Publication Data

Mark, Saralyn.
Stellar Medicine, A Journey Through the Universe of Women's Health — 1st ed.
p. cm.

1. Health. 2. Health—Women's Health I. Mark, Saralyn
Fiction, I. Title.
ISBN-13: 978-1-883283-78-0, Trade Paper
Copyright © 2011 by Saralyn Mark, M.D.

December 2011

DEDICATION

I dedicate this book to Idella (Bobbie) Mark—my wise mentor, my harshest critic, my treasured friend, my spectacular mother—her spirit lives on in all who loved her.

PREFACE

I have worked in the lofty halls of government, the corridors of chaotic emergency rooms, corporate offices and in medical school classrooms. All of this has given me a unique perspective on how and why we make decisions that affect the delivery of healthcare for women. This view allows me to share with you the most recent information in women's health, especially on sensitive issues, as well as what is coming in the future.

Every year I have a speaking schedule that takes me across the globe, where I present ideas and opinions to a wide audience and get feedback in return. I have talked to countless women across the world and watched certain answers send ripples of interest through the crowd. I've heard the laughter of self-recognition and seen faces open up with relief and hope. This book grew from my journey. The stories that I share with you chronicle my experiences facing challenging and often controversial issues in medicine so not every topic in women's health will be presented.

I've spent much of my career in women's health trying to cut through confusion and fear and find the simple solution to a problem. I've seen these emotions when it comes to how women react to medical information, whether it comes from their own doctor, a magazine article or a close friend. I speak with thousands of women each year. When I look out at an audience, I'm reminded of these basic truths; we experience the same issues, we want answers, and we want to understand how to keep ourselves healthy.

From my audiences, patients, and family, I've learned that in most cases, if we can take a deep breath, move beyond our fear, use our common sense, and work with the available science, we get somewhere. Sometimes the first step—taking a deep breath—comes because of humor.

In that light, I'd like to share with you a few of my experiences in women's health—the serious issues and the funny stories, and see if together we can work toward a better way. I believe that humor heals and opens us up to receiving messages. I have found that these stories, while sometimes funny, illustrate important and powerful messages for women's health. I have shared many of them in my travels and have found that this is what my patients, audiences or peers remember and they are then able to connect the story to the underlying health message.

This book offers a framework of science and experience to encourage you to live a balanced life and to help you maintain wellness even in the face of stress and trouble. It also encourages you to ask questions, to examine facts, and to think before reacting in fear. This book contains my advice based upon scientific evidence and explains the social and political environment shaping this information. Use it as a guide to help you make good decisions. These are my views and do not represent the views of organizations that I have advised over the years.

What has been frustrating for me as a doctor, and I know for you as a patient, is that there is never enough time to ask questions and get the answers that you need and deserve. So think of this book, as you read it as our time together, as doctor and patient, but in the comfort of your home.

Table of Contents

INTRODUCTION
—"I'm not your damn intern!"

"I'm not your damn intern!" I never thought that I would hear those words. You can imagine how shocked I was to hear my mother's doctor tell me that over the phone when I just asked him a few questions. The evening was March 17, 2008 at 7 pm. The reason why I know that time to the exact moment was the phone rang just as I was turning on the television set to catch the news on NBC.

"Sara, this is Dr. X., your mother has..."

At first, I remember thinking why is he using my first name and he gets to be a doctor when he is actually younger than I am. From the start I knew there was going to be an imbalance in the conversation. I told him that I could not hear what he just said and I wanted to turn my TV off. He then said it again—

"Your mother has pancreatic cancer."

I remember feeling like I had just been punched in the stomach. I could barely breathe. In a trance, I walked to the bench by the window in the living room and sat down. At that instant, I transformed from a shocked daughter to a doctor and to an advocate who was going to fight for my mother. This was the same doctor who had put my mother in a hospice in Denver two years before when she had broken her hip and had pneumonia. I live in Washington, D.C. and had to trust that the information he was giving me at the time was correct and the decision was appropriate. As we see with the gift of time, I came to learn that it was not an accurate assessment. This time, I was not going to sit idly by and believe everything I was told.

"How do you know that she has pancreatic cancer—do you have a path specimen?"

He said, "I have a CT scan and it shows a mass in the pancreas and the location makes it impossible to get a biopsy."

"Do you have any lab tests such as amylase levels, liver function tests, bio-markers—anything?"

It was then that he told me, "I am not your damn intern."

These were the wrong words to tell me at that moment. All I wanted at that instant was to now get off the phone and get to my mom. I reminded him that he had called me. He had just given my mother a death sentence and there was no reason to continue our conversation. I wanted to tell him something else, but I knew that was not going to help my mother get better medical care.

We all have moments that sear our minds. We remember where we were when the planes hit the World Trade Center or perhaps when our President was shot or elected. These times transform our lives if we can learn from them and not run away from the pain, sorrow or high emotions that surround them.

I also believe that there are no real coincidences and that the universe provides us what we need if we are receptive. I found that to be the case the night of March 17. Minutes after I got off the phone call, girlfriends from my gym arrived at my home. I had planned to have a dinner party that night to bring the "gym girls" together. I had just returned from Southeast Asia and wanted to talk about my exciting trip with them so I had arranged the dinner at my house. This was a group of five women; ages ranged from 30s to 50s and from very different backgrounds. Some were married, some with children, all worked in various careers from finance to art to politics.

Since my arrival to Washington, D.C. in 1995, I would go with them to the same gym class—a body conditioning class, every Saturday morning when I was in town. We would work out together and then have lunch at the same restaurant across the street, ordering salads and talking for at least an hour afterwards. As it often is with women, we felt a sisterhood connection. No issue was taboo for us to discuss. Over an hour, we would talk about our relationships, world events, movies, health issues from hot flashes to sex to back surgery, and, of course, politics. Sometimes these conversations were serious and other times filled with laughter and even tears. We often joked that we could be the characters in a new "Sex in the City" movie. So you can imagine how relieved I was to see them at my doorstep after my world had just collapsed.

I was in a state of shock when I told them very flatly that my mom had cancer, and I even had a bit of righteous anger when I relayed my conversation with her doctor. They listened, they hugged me, and then I cried. I could see in their eyes their love and concern. Calmly, they helped me piece together what I needed to do. This was just like all our conversations that we would have after the gym-sharing information, giving advice and knowing that we would have support if anything went wrong. With a new determination, I left the dinner table and went to my bedroom to call my family. While I was upstairs, they cleaned up and quietly left.

I tell this story because I want you to feel as you read this book that we are sitting around a table talking to each other and being open to new ideas and perspectives. I know that it can be difficult and sometimes impossible to cut through the debris and confusion to understand what is happening in the medical system as it affects your life and others. As you can see from my story, it can even be challenging for a doctor who has lots of knowledge and experience to get straight answers.

At times, the system even seems to foster this haze. For the most part, I don't think that it is intentional but built into an archaic system where hierarchy maintains control and roles. For example, in my phone call, I was clearly from the start not viewed as a peer but a patient or—worse yet—a family member of a patient. I was going to be told what was only necessary. I did not accept that boundary and it created an imbalance and hence hostility. All too often, patients are placed in that position and it leads to bad care.

Just as one was considered "un-American" to question why we were going to war with Iraq, I found that the health policies created during the first part of the 21st century were fostering an increasingly hostile environment as well. Women and girls were not able to get full information about reproductive healthcare and the public was bombarded with exaggerated tales of impending doom from bio-weapons and terror tactics. I cannot imagine that any portion of our society could be immune from all that fear, anger and paranoia—cardinal emotions of our generation at the turn of this new century.

In July 2006 I decided to resign my government position. The final straw for me was when President Bush vetoed stem cell research and signed his veto at the White House that month, surrounded by infants who were the progeny from "embryo adoption" programs. I had worked on these "adoption" programs when my office was asked to chair a work group to implement this new legislation. Millions of dollars went into these programs and we could not use the words "embryo donation" only "embryo adoption" to describe this issue.

I recall during the first few meetings, I asked the then Assistant Secretary of Health some questions about adoption of older children and was told that was not the role of the federal government. More of my questions were met with looks of dismay. Of course, I was not invited back to future meetings which was a relief until I saw the "embryo adoption" program advertised at the White House event. I knew at that moment that I could no longer do my work for the Department of Health and Human Services (DHHS). I now felt that I could do more in the private sector. Again, it was an issue of balance—the good no longer balanced the bad. However, I was going to greatly miss working with my colleagues—individuals who gave it their all to try to improve the lives of girls and women across the globe.

After I left, I formed SolaMed Solutions, LLC which allowed me to provide advice and guidance to the private sector and even to the government but with an ability to speak my mind. The first time that I gave a speech and did not feel restricted was liberating. I would have more moments like that in the future. Over the years, I had been asked to write a book, especially by my audiences, but I did not feel that I could until I left government and had the freedom to say what I believed to be important and true. As I think back, the draft titles of this book reflected my inner spirit at various points in time since my resignation from the DHHS.

At first, I wanted to call the book, *Sex, Chocolate, Wine and Shopping*. Again, it was probably because sex was so demonized over the years especially if it was not within the confines of a heterosexual marriage. I wanted to show that pleasure was actually good for health and to provide scientific evidence to support that principle. Then, I wanted to call it *Truth or Chocolate* after the fear generated around avian influenza or the bird flu outbreak and all the myths surrounding public health. This was followed by the furor over abstinence education, and I thought that a good title might be *Ms. Conception* which would allow me to discuss reproductive health. And then finally *Stellar Medicine: A Journey Through the Universe of Women's Health*.

I believe that my views, not just from inside of the beltway surrounding Washington D.C., but also from my own journey, especially during 2008, could help others. 2008 was a year that transformed my life in ways that were impossible to imagine. Everyday was a challenge to find balance. From a journey filled with pain and sadness, to sheer elation and to a deeper understanding about the connection between all of us on this planet, I felt that I was ready to write this book and to incorporate the sensational and controversial issues illustrated by the prior book titles into chapters.

I must admit when the ball dropped in Times Square on December 31, 2008, it was not a moment too soon—actually it even had an extra second to it which fit the year! Every month in 2008 was filled with something extraordinary—some years are like that. You have to hang on for dear life, but you know it will not be boring.

In early January 2008, I had gone to New Hampshire to work in the Democratic primary. The cold days walking from house to house, attending town halls and breathing the excitement of new ideas inspired me. At the end of January, I attended a gala in New York City for Virgin Galactic—the commercial space tourism venture of Sir Richard Branson. This was the beginning of the new space age and I was excited to see a part of it.

In February, I went to Thailand, Vietnam, Cambodia and a quick stop in China. It was to be a fun adventure with a former colleague from the Centers for Disease Control and Prevention (CDC). Unfortunately, she fell an hour before we were to begin our tour and I had to go on without her. What would have been 2 weeks filled with laughter and humor became a fact-finding mission. I really saw the impact of poverty, disease and stigma on these cultures. From a bird flu pandemic in Vietnam, an outbreak of hemorrhagic fever in Cambodia, the sex trade and child trafficking in Thailand and poor sanitation and pollution in China, I came away again transformed and ready to do something to make a difference.

Shortly after I returned in March, I felt the need to write a blog about the trip and to suggest ways to help these communities. I purchased a water well for a village in Cambodia and recommended to others that this was an ideal gift to give. However, a week later, my life was flipped upside down. My father was hospitalized with a heart condition, my mother was diagnosed with inoperable pancreatic cancer and a family member put himself back into active military duty despite being injured during a previous tour in Afghanistan. I felt that there was no safe haven. Instinctively, I turned more inward to search for my faith and belief in a compassionate universe.

From the end of March to early September, I was going back to Colorado to care for my parents who had frequent hospitalizations, and trying to keep my career intact amidst an economic crisis that our country had not experienced since the Great Depression. Looking back, it was the simple pleasures in life such as planting flowers, shopping for sale items, going for a hot fudge sundae with my mom, and having a glass of wine with a friend that kept me in balance. At times I felt that I was living in two worlds—one that was strictly professional and fully compartmentalized and another where I needed to remind myself to eat, sleep and breathe—basic survival at its best where adrenalin was the fuel to keep me going.

As I began September, I knew that I wanted to get back into the campaign. I was asked to serve on the Obama Health Care Advisory Committee joining colleagues from around the nation who shared the same commitment. I began to write again—this time, it was blogs, editorials and letters for leading newspapers.

It was invigorating to write about issues that were controversial and to engage the public in dialogue. At times, it was frightening to get angry responses about my views on reproductive health and how religion and policy are a dangerous marriage. But it was also encouraging to find so many enlightened individuals who were concerned about the travesty of our healthcare system, especially for women, and who had a desire to improve the lives of those who did not have a voice.

Yes, 2008 was quite a year. I just shared with you some of the peaks and valleys and there were many. I had to find my inner balance to stay afloat, but in the process, I gained some valuable insights.

After practicing medicine on Earth and in space, I want to share with you the adventures and health challenges of space travel to illuminate the daily experiences of living on this planet. Taking this universal perspective can embolden us to see the world of healthcare in a new light—from mundane to controversial issues that we frequently confront.

Many moons ago, I was someone's intern. Now, I want to be your doctor and help guide you on your life's journey filled with good health, wellness, and of course stellar medicine.

CHAPTER ONE
A PANDEMIC OF MISINFORMATION
—Truth or Consequences

"The moment we begin to fear the opinions of others and hesitate to tell the truth that is in us, and from motives of policy are silent when we should speak, the divine floods of light and life no longer flow into our souls."

—Elizabeth Cady Stanton

Politics is never far from one's life in Washington, D.C., but if you work for the government specifically, the way I did for over eleven years, you find that political winds blow directly through the office doors and affect everything from the way one approaches the work, to the vocabulary one uses to talk about it. I worked in Washington, D.C. through the Clinton and much of the Bush Administrations and continued to do so in the Obama years as a consultant. I am still amazed by how the character of the person leading the nation from the White House shapes the culture, the work ethic, and even the type of employees hired in the capital city. Even in the world of science, which should have immunity from shifting cultural opinions, politics affects both the tone and dissemination of the information at hand. Never is that more true than when a crisis hits.

When I think about a pandemic of misinformation, my mind immediately travels back to September 11, 2001. It was a perfect late summer day in Washington, D.C. Not only was the weather great, it was a big morning for me. I woke up early, excited for the day to begin. I worked at the Department of Health and Human Services (DHHS) at the time and we had been working for nearly six years preparing a massive osteoporosis and national bone health campaign. The press conference launching our program was scheduled for that morning. I was on my way in, passing through the section of the city near the State

Department, when I saw crowds of people running down the street in a panic. A man passed me carrying a small television.

"They collapsed," he said, meaning the towers.

He showed me the picture but the screen was so small I could only see a dust cloud on the screen. My phone rang. It was my assistant who was already at the office.

"Oh, God," she said. I'll never forget the way her voice cracked. "A plane hit the Pentagon. They say one is heading to the White House or to the Capitol near our office."

I took a deep breath and told her to leave the office and walk home. She did not argue with me.

While I was still talking to her, I looked around. It is hard to do justice to that moment in history. I can tell you that I watched a car slowly, almost carefully, roll over a curb and drive down the sidewalk. I walked by a hotel that was sealed off with yellow hazard tape. I understand they had received a bomb threat soon after the first plane hit. All the patrons had been escorted across the street to a small park. A waiter in pristine white gloves was serving tea to the evacuated guests, pouring it out of an ornate silver teakettle. It reminded me of the scene from the movie, Titanic, in which an orchestra played as the ship was sinking.

As soon as I hung up, I heard the rumors spreading across the crowd like a brush fire.

"A plane is heading for the White House."

"The Metro is going to be bombed."

"People have been killed at the Washington Monument."

These statements were made as if proven fact. It was impossible to know for sure what the truth was at that point. That was the start of a massive "pandemic of misinformation."

Everything happened so fast from there. The next minute, I was off running toward George Washington University Hospital, in full doctor mode. Not sure how severe the attack on the city was, I assumed the hospital would need all the help it could get. When I arrived, the doors were barred. I remember a huge crowd of people trying to get in.

A guard appeared at the front entrance. I showed him my government credentials and explained that I was a doctor and wanted to help. He cracked the door open and I slid inside. The hospital was in a total lock-down.

They gathered us all in the cafeteria on the second floor. Dozens of doctors and other medical professionals had arrived to help in what we all assumed was going to be a large-scale emergency crisis. The staff at the hospital interviewed each of us, asking about our skill sets and, in essence, triaging their resources.

We spent the day waiting for a rush of patients that never came. The attack on the Pentagon was such that the injured were severely burned and sent to a burn unit at another hospital. While I waited, though, I saw images of the attack for the first time on a big television screen in the cafeteria. I remember my muscles tightening up. It was a highly visceral reaction that I will never forget.

I can still see the faces of the people around me in that moment. The doctor sitting next to me had just arrived at Reagan National Airport to attend a medical conference, but took a taxi instead to George Washington University Hospital after the first plane hit. He had flown in from New York City. A female medical student in the room wore a hijab headscarf. She was also from Manhattan and scared to death for all of the people she knew back home. I remember thinking, even then, that her life had changed, and not just because she was from New York. I knew the fear that would spread across the country. No matter how sad it made me, I knew that she would be a symbol of that fear simply because of her religious beliefs.

In the end, not much happened at the hospital. I left around six that evening and boarded a Metro heading home. There were only a handful of people on the train. Everyone aboard that evening talked to each other. We all made eye contact. In a strange way, the attack brought us closer together.

When I got home, I sat in my house. It was quiet and I tried to relax as much as I could. Within minutes, I heard a fighter jet scream over the house, leaving Andrews Air Force Base on patrol. Needless to say, I ratcheted back to the press conference I had been so excited about on the morning of September 11, 2001. It became an afterthought, really. Everything did.

* * *

As with so many aspects of American life, my work place changed on September 11, 2001. That day there was a pandemic of misinformation that caused terrible fear. That, in turn, affected peoples' behavior. Rumors left people with no idea what was going to happen next. They did not even have reliable information on what had already occurred.

What surprised me then, and what has begun to preoccupy me since, is how the tone of fear that grew in 2001 has not abated, but instead increased. Not just fear of further attacks or fear of bioterrorism, but fear of natural or manmade weapons of mass destruction, of betrayals and situations spinning out of control. Increasingly since 2001, the tone surrounding us has been one of fear coupled with multiple warnings and words of caution.

Until 2009, one result of this fear (real or imagined) within the scientific community had been increasing limitations on what one said and wrote, and what programs we could develop. Decisions were not always based on science and evidence. Rather than an atmosphere where all ideas were encouraged and entertained, the conversation had narrowed. That's what happens when fear drives information rather than science. I believe fear starts at the top, moves through different governmental agencies, gets conveyed to the public, and ultimately affects an individual's behavior.

Living in a constant state of fear for a community certainly isn't healthy. On an individual level, it's not healthy either. Fear causes a person's adrenal glands to secrete hormones such as cortisol into the bloodstream to prepare the body for fight or flight. When the body gets the message that danger is near, the heart rate increases, pupils dilate, blood is diverted from the core to the legs, there is a suppression of the immune system and blood sugar levels rise. All of these things increase the risk of illnesses such as diabetes and heart disease. It's not in our best interest to be motivated by fear.

Although fear is often the natural, uncontrollable emotion following a public health scare, many times we respond to fear with radical shifts in behavior instead of thoughtful ones. September 11, 2001, was an obvious event with immediate, cataclysmic consequences. More often than not, other public health issues are more subtle. Nevertheless, warnings are often broadcast in such a dire tone that people feel compelled to immediately change the way they live. What concerns me is the science behind the warning often gets completely left behind while the average citizen ends up making a lifestyle change that may or may not be warranted. I've been interested in how the environment of fear influences the way we live. When are we going to start looking behind the scenes to examine the evidence and make our own decisions? When will we wake up and ask questions instead of just accepting what we hear?

How does this undertone of fear get disseminated in a community and then ultimately drive the way we live, sometimes in spite of scientific evidence to the contrary? I've also asked myself why health and terror scares seem to multiply in the fall, and what's the motive behind them? Could it possibly be related to elections and the need to get support from a populace that wants its leaders to do everything possible to keep them safe even if that means going to war or to take medications to fight deadly biological enemies?

When I hear about a public health warning such as the anthrax scare that followed 9/11, I'm learning to ask what is going on at the time. I now look at the political climate, the global landscape, and what reasons someone might have to distract me with fear of a disease. The anthrax scare was a good example of this. It erupted just as we started bombing Afghanistan, and it caused a major shift in our behavior. People were primed after the terrorist attacks against the World Trade Center and the Pentagon. Thousands of people went on Ciprofloxacin (Cipro) as a precaution against anthrax. People flocked to the doctor to get Cipro, taxing the medical system at a time when patients had legitimate colds and the flu.

In fact, the residuals of this fear are still with us—outliving the actual biological weapon. Although the individual, a government employee, who was supposedly responsible for sending anthrax-laden mail, has died, we still irradiate our government letters. I get mail in my NASA office that has been so baked; the letters crinkle like Rice Krispies when I open them. Sometimes I can hardly read them because the pages are sealed together. One year, I received my Christmas cards on Valentine's Day after they went through the irradiation process. As a nation we went along hook line and sinker with the anthrax scare, forgetting about what else was going on in the world, and obediently taking medication. In retrospect, our reaction was out of proportion to the scare.

This level of fear continued for several years after the events of 2001. Politicians appealed to this emotion in their campaigns for public office. Campaign ads depicted their candidates as strong protectors of the security of Americans against a backdrop of buildings collapsing. More importantly, for a time, it assuaged the public's potential misgivings for military actions in Iraq. "Pre-emptive strike" became a part of our lexicon to save America from further attacks.

Another example of the politics of fear is how the nation responded to reports of avian influenza or bird flu. Look at the political climate when that scare spread through the population. We were in a constant state of fear as the death rates increased in Iraq and Hurricane Katrina had just devastated communities along the coasts of Louisiana and Mississippi. Our President at the time was under criticism for how he handled both issues. I am not saying that the White House generated the bird flu issue—propagating the disease throughout the world. It did, however, very little to calm the public and ease their fears. If there was any silver lining in all of this it was that more funds and resources were directed towards building up the public health infrastructure and communities were encouraged to create plans and enhance their communication and outreach strategies during a public health crisis. The timing of all of this was quite interesting. For years, the Department of Health and Human Services had been quietly working on these plans. Now there was massive media frenzy where the public would be engulfed in a pandemic that could leave people dying in the streets with blood pouring from every orifice similar to what was seen in the pandemic of 1918-1919.

When the bird flu stories started to appear in the news, people reacted with near panic, hoarding the anti-viral drug, Oseltamivir (Tamiflu), which was needed for the general population at risk for seasonal flu. This left many communities without this medication to prevent or treat the flu which kills over 37,000 Americans each year—mostly young children and the elderly. The bird flu scare is another example of fear overrunning the science. In order to have sustained transmission of bird flu in the human environment, several genetic mutations would be required, but this message was often overlooked. Meanwhile, the country was terrified for a time, and again taxed the medical system needlessly.

When we hear about the next new virus or poison or even policy we need to see what else is going on in the world. Are people deliberately putting out messages to distract us from another issue? When Senator Edward Kennedy passed away in 2009, it set up a special election for his vacated seat in January 2010. Democrat Martha Coakley looked as if she would win, but she lost to Scott Brown, a Republican, for the seat that was held by Senator Kennedy for over 40 years. Many pundits claimed that fear over new healthcare legislation was a driving factor to this election—a bit of irony in that the driving passion of Senator Kennedy was health care reform.

For example, people were afraid that with new legislation, they would lose their existing healthcare coverage, their rates would increase and "Big Brother" would take over their lives and destroy one of the best healthcare systems in the world. One of the more egregious pieces of misinformation was that euthanasia or death squads for the elderly would be the norm. People became afraid that if grandma or grandpa was ill, the government would not allow them medical care and they would be left to die. In fact, the proposed legislation was just providing coverage for doctors to discuss end-of-life issues in a humane and compassionate manner. Interestingly, Scott Brown said that he would veto senate legislation on health care reform, although he had voted to support reform in Massachusetts. Many of the provisions in the senate bill had elements that were similar to the state bill.

The Administration and our health officials did not communicate well to the public about the need and benefits for health care reform. The positive components that most people would like such as removing pre-existing conditions, providing portability, creating healthcare exchanges where groups of people could negotiate for lower prices and covering preventive services in expanded community health centers were lost or overshadowed in the volatile debate. An atmosphere of fear and confusion predominated through the summer and fall of 2009 to the point where the public would rather accept the status quo that may not have worked for them, but at least they knew their enemy.

The Administration and the Democratic members of Congress did not fully appreciate the impact of some of the psychological and social factors in the nation during the time of the policy discussions on health care reform. People were afraid—they were scared that they would not have money for food or for their mortgages. The nation was in debt and this sense of financial ruin plagued the mindset and the behavior of the public. Delayed gratification for a healthcare bill that would not fully be implemented until four to five years from the time it was passed was simply not acceptable. The public got lost in the debate about the minutiae of a 2000 page bill and how much it would cost them as well as their children down the road. The potential cost-savings from reform did not resonate in the hearts or minds of the taxpayer. While at the same time, the Republicans understood the concerns of the public and how to use it to their advantage—it was political theater at the most dramatic level. We cannot ignore the fact that the United States desperately needs health care reform. Beyond the partisan wrangling, we have elected officials who need to represent the highest needs of their constituents and work together to achieve this goal.

While the debate on health care reform raged through most of 2009, there was another health story that occupied the news and the efforts of the government—the "Swine Flu." Even the name is example of misinformation. The correct nomenclature for the virus is H1N1 influenza, but for the first few months of this new infection, the media and the public responded to the much more visceral name "swine flu." Many early reports characterized H1N1 as a novel mutation, a new super virus that would sweep across the world, decimating the population. Memories of the anxiety over bird flu caused the fear level in this country to rise dramatically.

I remember the moment when I first heard about H1N1 influenza. It was a quiet Saturday morning near the end of April 2009, when the news began to break about cases of people dying of a new infection in Mexico. This infection had all the hallmarks of a serious public health crisis: a novel virus, young people dying, and an infection spreading quickly through the population. After working on the public health response to SARS in 2003 and working through a potential bird flu pandemic in 2005, I had a feeling we were in for a wild ride.

Within days, shelves in stores were wiped clean of hand sanitizers, gloves and facemasks. Tamiflu, scarce during the early days of the bird flu outbreak in Asia, was now becoming hard to find again. The media began reporting on cases of H1N1 infection in the United States. The Centers for Disease Control and Prevention (CDC) started holding news conferences and teleconferences with doctors around the nation. We knew in the spring of 2009 that we were in the midst of a potential pandemic, and the severity and impact was hard to predict. With each new case, the level of fear began to grow. Talk about the 1918 "Spanish flu" increased just as we had seen when bird flu erupted into the news. Again, stories of how healthy people dropped dead within hours with blood oozing from their eyes and mouths just escalated our anxiety of what could be around the corner.

The funny or perhaps odd thing was that I never placed the nation's pandemic plan in my bookcase in my office at NASA. Instead I kept the giant binder on the floor next to my desk. Perhaps, it gave me a sense of confidence that we were ready for anything. The fascinating thing was that the plan was designed for an infection that occurred overseas such as in Asia. We were expecting bird flu not a homegrown variety from our own continent. The Vice President took a bit of flak in the early spring for suggesting that it may not be a good idea to take public transportation and to fly. He was actually correct according to our pandemic plan, but the challenge was that the virus had originated in North America. Social distancing as the Vice President was suggesting would have potentially worked if the virus had not yet spread widely—it would have helped to slow down the infection.

During the first few weeks and months of this new infection, I gave many briefings on H1N1 influenza to NASA and its occupational health clinics. NASA has always done an outstanding job tackling health emergencies that impact their employees—from the devastation of Hurricane Katrina in 2005 to the anthrax scare. As their medical consultant, I attended the White House Summit on Flu in June 2009 that was held at the National Institutes of Health (NIH). Leaders from the DHHS, Department of Homeland Security (DHS) and the Department of Education (DoE), as well as several governors and public health officials from every state were in attendance. Even the President participated from his meetings with the G-8 leaders in Italy. The need for a new vaccine and priority groups were extensively discussed as well as the importance of communication. Over and over again, it was stressed that public health officials needed to be upfront about what they knew and did not know—honesty and transparency were the buzzwords. Lessons from prior health debacles were not to be forgotten. The fine balance between causing fear and pandemonium and raising awareness and concern to generate constructive actions was emphasized.

Many of my concerns about women and children came to pass. We all expected that the fall would be a difficult time. We saw high infection rates when kids went to summer camp. In fact, some summer camps had to close after they became clinics for sick children and had quarantined most of their campers. We saw in the spring of 2009 that schools became hot beds for infections. Thousands of schools across the nation closed during the first few weeks of the infection in the spring. Although closing schools slowed down infection rates, it was also challenging for families as parents needed to work and some children got many meals at schools. So closing schools was not to be a first line tool, but teachers prepared for distance learning just in case.

I have always been concerned about women's responses to infection especially after having a harrowing experience when I was infected with a strain of influenza A that was not covered by the influenza vaccine in 2004. About three weeks after I received my flu shot that year, a NASA colleague came back from Antarctica quite ill after he was exposed to a flu outbreak at the South Pole. He tried to continue to work despite a hacking cough. A few days after being exposed to him, I suffered from a high fever, chills and a cough that never stopped. One day, I coughed so hard that I could actually hear a few ribs pop out of their cartilage support that had kept them connected to my sternum or breastbone. Now every time I took a breath, my own ribs stabbed my lungs. The pain was excruciating. I subsequently developed pneumonitis, bronchitis, and pharyngitis—it seemed as if every "itis" available belonged to me. After weeks of steroids—oral and inhaled, nebulizers, painkillers and even antibiotics for the secondary bacterial infection that developed, I finally began to heal.

I believe that I developed a cytokine storm—an immune/inflammatory response to an infection in my body. Cytokines are messengers for the immune system. I also believe that my immune system that had been healthy and competent to begin with was revved up by the flu shot that I received prior to my infection. It stimulated my immune system, but the antibodies did not completely attack the new virus that I was exposed to—a set up for a cytokine storm. Basically, my body was attacking itself trying to get rid of the virus or foreign invader—a form of "collateral damage" in military parlance.

In June 2008, I attended a conference In New Orleans, Louisiana sponsored by the Organization for the Study of Sex Differences. It was a gathering of scientists to evaluate sex and gender-based research. Dr. Sabra Klein from the Johns Hopkins Bloomberg School of Public Health gave a brilliant presentation on the immune reaction to yellow fever among male and female animals. Her findings were compelling, and I asked after her lecture if we could translate these findings to what we should do to protect women during a pandemic. Basically, her studies showed that female animals may be more resistant than males to yellow fever infection, but once they are infected they can mount a very robust inflammatory response. During that summer, I was working on NASA's plan for a bird flu pandemic. I wondered if her findings could be translated to influenza—thinking of my own prior experiences with the flu.

I simply asked, "If women may be more resistant to infection but once infected, they mount vigorous reactions, could we potentially use less vaccine to get an effective response?" If that was the case, we might be able to give women a smaller dosage of vaccine thus making more available. Perhaps, we could use the disadvantage to our advantage.

Researchers at Walter Reed Army Medical Center conducted and published a study in 2008 that showed women's responses to half doses of a seasonal flu vaccine were comparable to men's responses to a full dosage. Furthermore, women had more injection site and systemic reactions such as headaches, fatigue and muscle aches. These data are compelling. On the downside, if women mount robust inflammatory responses that could cause more secretions in the lungs, they were potentially at higher risk for developing pneumonia and Acute Respiratory Distress Syndrome (ARDS) which are potentially fatal complications. I also thought that pregnant women may lose their resistance to infections because their immune systems have changed so that they do not reject the fetus, yet they would still have a strong inflammatory response—a type of cytokine storm similar to what I experienced. It would also be harder to ventilate a pregnant woman because of the increased resistance and pressure on the lungs from her pregnancy. Additionally, more adipose tissue or fat during a pregnancy could lead to a greater inflammatory response since fat cells are a repository for inflammatory cells—a perfect storm for a medical disaster.

When H1N1 surfaced in Mexico in April 2009, I was interested to see if women had higher mortality rates. I contacted colleagues at CDC and asked for data. As I expected, there were higher mortality rates among women. Although some thought that this was due to decreased access to healthcare for women in Mexico, I believed that it was due to the inherent biological differences in immunity between men and women. Mexico does have a public health infrastructure and women do have opportunities to get care. Around mid May, the CDC was also reporting higher morbidity and mortality rates for women, especially among pregnant women in the United States. In fact, in just the first eight months of the H1N1 influenza pandemic, pregnant women had the highest hospitalization rates and 6% of all deaths although they represent only 1% of the U.S. population.

In May 2009, the CDC announced that pregnant women should be cautious. They recommended that if a pregnant woman was diagnosed with H1N1, she should start Tamiflu immediately. I shared my thoughts on the higher risk for women through NASA briefings and lectures at medical conferences, and in articles and blog entries. By spreading awareness, my colleagues and I felt we could help women be better prepared while promoting the need for more studies to explore the etiology behind these sex differences. Not surprisingly, there were some naysayers; I just let the data speak for itself.

The impact of sex hormones on the immune and inflammatory system is an important area to explore. It may have relevance not only to infectious diseases but also to other illnesses such as cardiovascular diseases and even cancer. By understanding these influences, better medical care can be provided. This can help alleviate the anxiety that is generated when we see differences in how men and women present when they are ill, but have not known what to do with these observations.

* * *

In the early days of the 2009 H1N1 influenza pandemic, pig farmers were very upset that the infection was called swine flu. They felt that it caused inappropriate fear illustrated by people refusing to eat pork. Even pigs were killed in some countries such as Egypt that all ready had some religious prohibitions against eating pork. Pigs have always been susceptible to both human and avian influenza and can act as a melting pot brewing new viruses in which the genes from birds, pigs and humans have re-assorted.

To put this into perspective, swine flu cases have been found in humans in the United States for decades. In 1976, an outbreak occurred in the United States. It began when 13 soldiers at Fort Dix were diagnosed with a new influenza strain and experienced severe respiratory symptoms. One soldier died. Public health officials deemed the virus to be similar to the 1918-19 pandemic. That outbreak killed 20 million worldwide.

At the time, the virus was confined to the military base. Fearing the worst, however, the government urged the public to get vaccinated. Even President Ford recommended vaccination. Shots started in October and by December, cases of Guillain-Barre syndrome began to manifest. Guillain-Barre is an autoimmune disorder in which the body's immune system attacks the nervous system. Often, it starts with weakness and tingling in the legs and progresses up the body, sometimes resulting in paralysis. Most sufferers recover fully, but the disease can be fatal.

Once people became ill from the vaccination, the government stopped them. At that point, nearly 40 million Americans had received the vaccine. The risk of developing Guillain-Barre was 1 in 100,000.

How the swine flu outbreak played out in 1976 is a perfect example of the pressures public health officials face. If they had erred on the side of prudence, and a pandemic like that which occurred in 1918 struck again, millions could have died. In the end, they protected the public, and their actions are now considered a "fiasco."

Keeping in mind the calamity from the pandemic of 1918 as well as the 1976 outbreak, public health officials prepared to deal with H1N1. At the same time, countries were trying to minimize the public reaction to H1N1 influenza. In the spring of 2009, there were efforts by China, Great Britain, Japan and other countries to caution the World Health Organization (WHO) against declaring the H1N1 outbreak a pandemic.

There is often confusion regarding the definition of a pandemic. The World Health Organization has a six-phase scale leading up to an outbreak becoming a pandemic. Phases one through three describe when a virus is predominately infecting animals and few humans are affected. Phase one is when the virus circulating among animals is not spreading to humans. Phase two is when a virus is spreading through an animal population and has caused infection in humans. This is when a potential pandemic is first identified. Phase three occurs when animals have passed a virus to humans in sporadic cases, but no human-to-human transmission has occurred. Phase four is reached when a virus sustains human-to-human transmission. Phase five is reached when human-to-human transmission of a virus has spread to at least two countries in one WHO region. The final stage, Phase six, is when a pandemic is declared. It is defined by community wide outbreaks of the virus in at least two WHO regions. Lacking in the definition is any discussion of the seriousness of the virus. A pandemic is simply a geographical definition of how a disease is spreading.

Many countries feared that the designation of this H1N1 outbreak as a pandemic could cause "worldwide panic and confusion." During the spring of 2009, there was a global recession and economic despair. Countries were concerned that a pandemic might stop people from traveling and spending money further hurting the economies of the world. Some of have wondered if these concerns influenced the WHO, and its Director General, Margaret Chan, to delay declaring a pandemic even though there were reports from many countries that the disease had spread. I recall hearing during the World Health Assembly at the WHO in May 2009 multiple reports of cases of H1N1 influenza in small and large countries around the world. Even the health ministers from the islands in the Caribbean were discussing their worries over having enough resources to take care of their citizens. I was also overhearing stories from scientists that the vaccine was not growing very well in cell culture. Representatives from around the world were nervous about several issues—from an impending economic catastrophe and a potential public health disaster when H1N1 hit their shores.

As one can imagine, the declaration of a pandemic should be a simple matter of fact. How can one caution against a factual declaration? In essence, the request by countries such as China and Great Britain was to change the definition. Their tenet seemed to be that although the disease spread quickly, it had not been severe enough to justify the label "pandemic."

What is the impact of declaring H1N1 a pandemic? The World Bank commissioned a study looking at the economic impact of avian flu. In a 2008 publication, this report specifically examined what effect a human influenza pandemic would have on the economy especially if humans had a limited immunity to the virus. In regard to mortality rates, the report cited a worst-case scenario of 180 to 260 million fatalities. Using low, mild and severe outbreaks, they estimated a reduction of the worldwide Gross Domestic Product (GDP) ranging from 0.7 to 4.8 percent. It was estimated that the cost of a severe pandemic could be as much as $3 trillion. That said, it is easy to see why some countries wanted to avoid labeling the H1N1 outbreak as a pandemic in these already troubled economic times.

Influenza viruses are unpredictable and each wave of a pandemic can be different. In the 1918 pandemic the first two waves were mild and then it came back with a vengeance and millions of people died around the world. The first two waves of the H1N1 flu pandemic resulted in nearly 17,000 American deaths with cases in over 212 countries. It was estimated that 18% of the population in the United States had been infected. But because more people had not died, nations around the world questioned whether H1N1 should have been declared a pandemic. Some began to ask whether it was a conspiracy of drug companies to make money from vaccines and anti-viral agents.

The WHO found itself in a lose/lose situation at the beginning of 2010. In January, 2010, the WHO came under fire for possibly succumbing to pressure when it finally decided to declare the outbreak a pandemic. The Parliamentary Assembly of the Council of Europe, a human rights advocacy group from France, asked the European Union to investigate the WHO's decision. The question likely sprung from the relatively low fatality rate of the disease. A WHO spokesman, Gregory Hartl, is quoted as saying, "A pandemic has nothing to do with severity or number of deaths. A pandemic literally is a global spread of a disease." Yet, this fact that had been issued from the time the pandemic was declared in June 2009 did not appease the public's perception of malfeasance.

During the beginning of this pandemic, there were a number of Internet rumors circulating in cyber-space about how a former senior government official was on the board of directors for the company that patented a popular anti-viral medication. In truth, the individual was on the board of directors and did continue to own stock in the company. As usual, the "rumor" was steeped in truth, but the pandemic declaration was not a publicity stunt to popularize anti-viral medication.

In a statement dated January 22, 2010, the WHO responded to claims that it created a "fake" pandemic to benefit drug companies. It cited the fact that the virus was confirmed to be different than other influenza viruses in the lab, early data showed person to person communicability, and data from Mexico showed that the disease could be fatal. Their statement provided the data they used when making their decision to declare a pandemic. In April, 2009, the WHO had confirmed cases in 9 countries. By June of that year, 74 countries had reported cases in more than two WHO regions. The definition for a pandemic had been more than met which I had actually thought had occurred as early as in May.

We also need to keep in mind that the healthcare systems in developed nations are stronger today than years ago. We should not expect to lose millions of people to diseases that we can prevent or treat. We do fear the day that there will be a "super virus" that has a high case fatality rate—basically killing everyone in its tracks. This is not a smart bug since it will eventually die with no more carriers to propagate it. However, we always need to stay vigilant and on guard to catch these agents early.

Response to the H1N1 flu vaccine in the fall of 2009 also shows just how hard it can be to manage the reality of healthcare within the larger picture of the media and public impression. Back in May 2009, the CDC assured the public that vaccines would be available by October. As the pandemic flu season escalated in the fall of that year with children going back to school, many areas did not have access to enough vaccine. As suspected in the spring, the virus was not growing well in cell cultures, thus taking more time than hoped to make the vaccine. People stood in lines and waited for schools to get vaccine for their children, but for some it did not arrive until late November and December. By then the patience of the public had been expended and the fear that this disease could kill them or their family members had largely subsided. Health departments had finally received enough vaccines, but they had difficulty generating interested patients.

After December 2009, case numbers decreased as was to be expected, By February 2010, over 70 million vaccines had been administered within the United States, and it was estimated that over 57 million Americans had been infected. So just with these facts alone, infection rates would be expected to go down. Additionally, waves of a pandemic generally last only a few months and then subside, but can come back with a vengeance as people who have no prior immunity to the virus become infected or the virus mutates and becomes more virulent. This is why the CDC and the WHO kept encouraging people to get vaccinated and maintain proper hand washing and hygiene.

Nearly 17,000 people died from H1N1 during the first eight months of the pandemic—most were under the age of 65, with over 1730 children in the United States. There were more than 260,000 Americans hospitalized which is probably an underestimate since not everyone who was hospitalized or died was tested. Yet, the public became complacent and no longer afraid of the new virus. I find this to be intriguing and concerning at the same time. I knew families of patients who died from this virus and their lives are forever scarred. To have lost even one person from a largely preventable cause is simply heartbreaking.

I remember spending hours in a hospital waiting room with the family of a healthy 53-year-old man who became ill while on a business trip to Denver. My mom was hospitalized in a room in the intensive care unit next to this man. I wanted to give hope to this family, but each day I could see the valiant efforts of the medical team failing. Then one day, I no longer saw the family in the waiting room and I learned that he had died. It touched me deeply that he would never know how brave his children were while they waited and prayed for him to recover and come home. This is one reason why it bothered me that rumbles began that the pandemic was a "fake."

Overall, I think that the CDC and the state departments of health did a good job to inform the public and to encourage vaccination and proper hygiene. Many hospitals treated patients quickly and efficiently with all the latest technology that was available. We can only imagine what the impact would have been without those measures. So in some ways, by people doing a good job and keeping the death rates low, the public became comfortable that the disease was not that bad. Ironically, I would rather see that outcome than what could have befallen us.

As one can see, public health scares are tempting tools in our troubled economic and political times. We can help to diminish some of that fear. We need to learn to ask more questions and think through the consequences of our actions rather than just reacting in fear. Ask yourself who is the messenger? What is their bias? What are the consequences?

The truth is that the human body adapts fairly well to its surroundings. Even bodies in space adapt to that environment within a few days. We are exposed to viruses and bacteria everywhere, but we don't always get infected and become ill because, most of the time, our immune systems can fight the attacks. What are we willing to tolerate and risk so that we are not driven by fear? Instead of panicking about unseen illnesses, in many ways we would be better served by taking a deep breath and going for a walk to get a clear perspective.

I often think back to September 11, 2001 as our lives have so dramatically changed. The fear we felt on that day was appropriate. For me, it led to a constructive behavior—rushing to George Washington University Hospital to see if I could help. For many of us, it brought our families closer together. In reality, it brought our entire country closer together for a time, just as it did with the few of us on the Metro that night. I believe it encouraged us to slow down our lives and appreciate what is most important to us.

At the same time, the fear generated by that day appeared to have been used by politicians to justify a declaration of war in Iraq based on incomplete information. It led to families losing loved ones overseas, some of whom came home in coffins and for those who survived the battles, to return home with "invisible injuries."

We need to learn to ask more questions and think through the consequences of our actions rather than just reacting in fear. In most cases, the healthiest thing we can do is NOT be afraid, but pay attention to basic common sense, sanitation, moderation and logic. Our bodies are designed for health, wellness and balance, and at some point we have to trust that, and not fall prey to fear.

How many of the health scares of the past few years have come to pass and how much time, medical resources and money were spent in preparing for them? When we look at this candidly, we find we would be better served by asking questions, evaluating the science and holding the government accountable for the information it generates and shares with the public. So much healthier to do this than allow fear to drive our behavior and prevent us from enjoying our lives.

Even in times of confusion during pandemics and other crises, we need to keep an open mind and ask thoughtful questions. Through honest communication and information, we can get through any event, including H1N1 influenza, the first real pandemic in this century.

Stellar Questions:

Can taking antiviral drugs hurt you?

An antiviral drug, particularly for the flu, decreases the ability of the virus to reproduce. This differs from a vaccine that builds the body's natural immunity to the virus, thus attempting to forestall infection. For treating the flu, an antiviral course should begin within two days after showing signs of illness. The medication can shorten the duration of the flu, and also help to avoid dangerous complications. Flu viruses can also develop resistance to these agents so appropriate use is important.

There can be side effects when taking antivirals. Zanamivir (Relenza) should not be taken by people who have underlying heart or respiratory illness since people have to inhale it. This includes asthma and chronic lung disease. Other side effects have been noted such as diarrhea, nausea, bronchitis and headaches. For Oseltamivir (Tamiflu), most side effects reported are gastrointestinal in nature. These include nausea and vomiting. Risk of experiencing these side effects can be reduced if taken with food.

Researchers have been looking into another concern of antivirals. According to one study, the drugs account for two to 15 percent of cases of acute renal failure. Antiviral medications mentioned in this study were Cidofovir, Adefovir, Dipivoxil, Tenofovir, and Acyclovir.

According to the CDC, Oseltamivir is the preferred antiviral for treating pregnant women. Both drugs recommended for treating H1N1 influenza, Oseltamivir and Zanamivir, can be taken by children. Oseltamivir is FDA approved for children over one year old. It can be prescribed for even younger children in cases of emergency. Zanamivir is approved for children seven years old and up, and should not be given to children with asthma. There have been cases of neuro-psychiatric complications in children so caution is necessary when giving these drugs to this group.

A new drug, Peramivir, was given emergency authorization for usage during the H1N1 influenza pandemic even though it was still in clinical trials and not tested in pregnant women. This drug can be given intravenously which sometimes is helpful when patients are intubated or using a breathing tube and cannot take medications orally. The drug may lower white blood cell counts that can impair one's ability to fight infections. As with any medication, there are risks and benefits that need to be measured.

Can taking the flu vaccine give me the flu?

Each year, a new flu vaccine is offered. It is produced using three viruses that have been circulating in the southern hemisphere during their winter. For the 2009 season, a separate vaccine was developed for the H1N1 influenza virus because it was too late to incorporate it into the seasonal flu vaccine.

There are two forms of the flu vaccine. One form, the flu shot, contains the dead virus. The second vaccine, the nasal spray, contains live virus that has been weakened. They do not cause the flu. Once the vaccine is given, antibodies develop in the body within three to four weeks.

According to the CDC, the flu shot cannot cause someone to contract the flu virus. The virus in the flu shot is dead, and tested to make sure it is dead before given out to patients. It is true, however, that some people are not protected from the flu after getting their shots. This may occur if they are exposed right after the shot because their bodies have not had time to develop immunity. There are also some people who do not respond effectively to the vaccine such as the elderly, young children or immune comprised patients.

The nasal spray, although it contains live virus, should not cause the flu either. It is not recommended for immune compromised patients or healthcare providers who see these patients since the virus used in the nasal spray is weakened but not dead. Interestingly, the virus is "cold-adapted," meaning it infects the cooler nasal passage but cannot infect the lungs.

What is the difference between seasonal and pandemic flu?

Every year, the flu spreads. This is called the seasonal flu. It follows a predictable pattern, with outbreaks usually in the winter months. This is the type of flu that scientists attempt each year to develop the most effective vaccine against. According to the CDC, five to 20 percent of the American population comes down with the flu annually. Each year, 200,000 are hospitalized and around 37,000 people die from the illness.

The 2009 H1N1 influenza was a new strain of flu that spread worldwide. The WHO declared it a pandemic in June 2009. This declaration is not necessarily about how deadly this new strain was, but that it spread across the globe. Such pandemic flu strains do not occur every year. In fact, they have only occurred three times in the 20th century.

A pandemic flu outbreak represents many challenges that the seasonal flu does not. First, we generally have developed some immunity to the seasonal flu from past exposure. Pandemic flu is a new strain and there are few pre-existing defenses against it. It also can occur and spread more rapidly, overwhelming vaccination attempts, availability of antiviral medications, and the medical infrastructure in general. They have the potential to cause a major impact on society.

What causes a novel flu virus?

There are two types of new flu strains: One, seen in the seasonal flu, is a slight variant of an existing strain. In other cases, however, drastically new flu viruses can emerge. These novel influenza viruses come about in a different way than the slight changes that happen each year to the seasonal flu.

Antigen drift is when an influenza virus slightly mutates producing changes in the viral proteins that help it to infect and replicate in a host's cells. It happens continuously, and results in the development of new strains of the flu. As the change occurs, usually one of the new strains becomes dominant. That dominant strain hangs around for a few years before it is replaced by a new strain. Antigen drift is why vaccines are updated each year.

Unlike drift, which is associated with the seasonal flu, antigen shift is associated with a pandemic flu. When a flu strain experiences significant genetic change in its surface proteins that allows it to even jump species this is called antigen shift. When this happens, the virus is so different that now we do not have prior exposure and immunity. Thus, it can spread much faster than a virus that simple drifted.

Should I worry about anthrax?

Anthrax is an infection caused by the bacteria, Bacillus anthracis. It is present in domesticated animals such as cattle and sheep. Therefore, it is more common in heavily agricultural areas. Most human exposures to anthrax come from people working with animals or on farms.

The symptoms of an anthrax infection vary based on how the disease develops. Most cases of infection enter the body through a cut in the skin. Such skin infections start out looking much like an insect bite. Over a few days, it becomes an ulceration with a necrotic, black center. The nearest lymph glands may swell. With treatment, death is rare.

Anthrax can also enter the body through inhalation. Symptoms might resemble those of a cold. Within a few days, severe breathing problems will occur. Inhalation anthrax is very dangerous and even with treatment; nearly half of those infected will die.

Finally, anthrax can also infect the intestines. This can occur when infected meat is eaten. The intestinal tract becomes very inflamed. Other symptoms include nausea, vomiting, fever, throat lesions and difficulty swallowing. It can be fatal.

There is a weapons grade anthrax that has been manipulated in the lab so that the particles are so fine that it is easily carried in the air and can be inhaled into the lungs causing disease. This is a form of biological warfare and was the type that was used in the 2001 anthrax attack. As we learned during that episode, some patients can survive if they are quickly treated with the appropriate antibiotics.

Can you feed a cold and starve a fever?

The old saying, "feed a cold and starve a fever," may have come from a time where physicians believed that colds were caused by the body temperature going down and fevers were caused by the body temperature going up. The saying may have come from the idea that you increase calories to warm the body back up and decrease the calories to cool the body off. When a person gets a bacterial or a viral infection, chemicals are released into the blood stream that stimulates the brain to increase the body temperature or a fever. This helps to make the body less hospitable to the infection.

Some researchers, however, see it differently. They looked at how food affects the immune system. After having subjects fast overnight, they gave one group a "liquid" meal of containing about 1,200 calories. The other group received the same volume of water. What they found was that the calories favored "cell-mediated immunity" whereas starvation favored a "humoral immune response." A humoral immune response involved the body creating antibodies, whereas cell-mediated immunity involves T lymphocytes, a type of white blood cell. The body when fighting viruses uses both types. However, researchers feel that calories stimulate one immune response and starvation stimulates another. Thus, the concept of feeding a cold and starving a fever could be more than just an old wives' tale. Nonetheless, it is important to maintain good nutrition when you are ill. No one would recommend starvation.

Why are the elderly and young more susceptible to complications from the seasonal flu virus?

The very young under the age of two and the elderly over the age of 65 are at a higher risk of developing serious complications from the seasonal flu virus. These groups are more at risk of life-threatening respiratory issues developing if they contract the flu virus. Another factor these groups face is the state of their immune system. For the young, they have not built up an immune response to the virus yet. For the elderly, their immune systems are declining naturally as they age.

According to the CDC, the flu shot is very effective in helping the elderly survive the seasonal flu. For the older population that is not living in a chronic-care facility, the seasonal vaccine is 30-70 percent effective in preventing pneumonia and influenza. For those living in a facility, the effectiveness is 50 to 60 percent, and the vaccine has been found to be 80 percent effective in preventing death from the flu. Infants under six months are particularly at risk, for they are too young to be vaccinated but are also prone to severe complications if they contract the virus. The CDC strongly recommends that household members be vaccinated to lessen the child's exposure.

For H1N1, however, things may be a little different. Elderly individuals may need higher vaccine doses to mount an effective immune response. Early in 2009, the CDC studied whether our older population had antibodies that could help protect them from H1N1 influenza already in their blood. The idea is that the population may have been exposed to a similar virus decades ago.

One study looked at the cases of H1N1 in California from April 23 to August 11, 2009. During that period, 1,088 patients were hospitalized with the virus. The median age of those hospitalized was 27, and 68 percent of 1,088 had risk factors for seasonal flu complications. Thirty-one percent of the people required intensive care. Eleven percent died and the majority of whom were over 50 years old.

From these results, the researchers posited that the median age was younger than with seasonal flu. Infants had the highest rate of hospitalization. So, although younger people seemed to be getting seriously sick from the virus, older people were still more at risk of developing a fatal complication probably because of other co-morbid conditions.

Can dead bodies cause illnesses?

On January 12, 2010, a quake measuring 7.0 on the Richter scale devastated Haiti. It severely damaged the infrastructure of the island and resulted in a significant loss of life with corpses rotting in the streets. Due to that, many people feared that corpses would intensify the public health catastrophe by spreading disease.

According to the Funeral Consumers Alliance, this is not true. This myth developed when some morticians told customers that they must embalm a family member's body so that it will not contaminate the groundwater.

In January 2010, the WHO released a report specifically on the situation in Haiti. They stated "corpses do not represent a public health threat." In the case of Haiti, death was usually due to trauma from the Earthquake, not disease. However, infection prevention was recommended for those in direct contact with the corpses.

What is the difference between a cold and flu?

Viruses that affect the respiratory system in humans cause both the common cold and the flu. Although the symptoms of the two illnesses can be very similar, the viruses are different. Sometimes, it can be very difficult to tell the two apart.

As a rule of thumb, the flu is worse than the common cold. Symptoms of the flu include body aches, fever, fatigue, and cough. Often, colds show themselves as runny or stuffed noses. Colds are less likely to cause serious complications.

As the name would imply, the common cold is far more common. According to the CDC, 22 million school days are missed per year due to the cold. Children can have upwards of ten colds a year.

It should be added that what is commonly called the "stomach flu" is not a flu at all. Influenza generally does not cause gastrointestinal symptoms although H1N1 influenza was occasionally associated with vomiting and diarrhea. Many other viruses, such as rotaviruses, noroviruses and sapo-viruses, can cause what people call the stomach flu. Parasites and bacteria can cause gastrointestinal symptoms as well.

Why should you not take antibiotics when you have a viral infection?

Antibiotics treat bacterial infections. Bacteria are found naturally all over our bodies and can cause illness. Often, illnesses caused by bacteria will not get better until antibiotics are taken.

Viruses, on the other hand, are even smaller than bacteria. They cannot live outside of the body's cells and can cause illnesses such as the common cold and the flu. Antibiotics have no effect on viruses at all.

The danger of overusing the medication is antibiotic resistance. If you take antibiotics for an illness that they cannot treat, such as a viral infection, they may not work when you do need them to fight a bacterial infection. It is thought that the appearance of antibiotic resistance bacteria, some call them super-bugs, was caused by the overuse of antibiotics.

Does prior exposure to seasonal flu weaken responses to H1N1 or pandemic flu?

During the pandemic, healthy middle-aged adults were harder hit compared to infants or older individuals which is just the reverse with what happens with seasonal flu infections. One hypothesis is that pre-existing antibodies in middle-aged adults recognized the 2009 H1N1 virus, but attacked lung tissue rather than stopped the H1N1 infection. These malfunctioning antibodies developed after the body was exposed to seasonal flu in the past. They recognized the H1N1 virus as foreign and attacked it but then the complex of antibody and H1N1 virus infiltrated the lungs and stimulated the cytokine pathway or chemical messengers to promote inflammation and damage lung tissue. This is called the "original antigenic sin."

Studies need to be conducted in animals to confirm this mechanism and to determine if there are sex differences showing whether more women are impacted. Additionally, research into whether prior flu vaccines can stimulate antibodies to do this with viruses that don't perfectly match up such as giving a pandemic flu shot and being exposed to seasonal flu virus or vice versa. Also, this could be an issue with seasonal flu vaccines that don't completely match the seasonal flu strains that are circulating that year. It is a complex situation that needs to be further understood in order to best treat it. For example, one treatment could inhibit the formation of these antibody-viral complexes.

Why did women have more complications and die more often from H1N1 influenza?

Women may have robust immune responses that may account for the higher incidence rates of auto-immune diseases. They may initially be more resistant to infection compared to men, but pregnant women may lose that resistance to protect the fetus from rejection. Thus, they may be more susceptible to infection. They may, however, still be capable of mounting a vigorous inflammatory response resulting in a cytokine storm and possible lung damage. In addition, the impact of elevated sex hormones such estrogen, progesterone, or testosterone on the cardiovascular system during pregnancy increases complications. Estrogen is associated with expanding blood vessels (vasodilatation) that could worsen complications such as shock caused by H1N1. Studies are needed to evaluate the impact of sex hormones on treatments such as Tamiflu.

CHAPTER TWO
HAIR DYE AND THE KILLER BRA
—Medical Myths and the True Story

> *Doubt thou the stars are fire;*
> *Doubt that the sun doth move;*
> *Doubt truth to be a liar;*
> *But never doubt I love.*

—William Shakespeare, *Hamlet*

Sally Ride, first American woman in space, was interviewed frequently before her historic flight in 1983. For years after her first trip out of our atmosphere, she tried to avoid the media. It was easy to see why she might want to. Male astronauts aren't asked questions such as, "will you cry when things go wrong," or "do you plan to have children." My favorite question she was asked was whether she needed to wear a bra in space.

"There is no sag in zero-g," she answered.

It is easy to see from her interaction with the media how easy myths, as well as stereotypes, have the legs they have. All women do not cry when things go wrong, not even in space. Nor are women so delicate that everyone's first concern should be about potential fertility.

Ironically, we've given these types of myths a name that makes many women cringe. We call them "old wives' tales." It is a saying that can be dated all the way back to ancient Greece. Even in our times of rising political correctness, the label has endured regardless of its age and gender stereotyping.

No matter who you are or how you've been raised, it's so easy to fall into believing these tales without looking into the truth. I vividly remember a time in my childhood where the blurry line between truth and tale came to our door, or rather out of it. I was two years old and loved being an escape artist—climbing out of my crib and strollers. It got to a point that my mom would put bells on my shoes to keep a handle on me. One time I even escaped from the dryer that my brother put me in.

On one very cold day in Denver, I slipped out the front door. I almost froze outside before my parents found me on the front step. I found that it was much easier to push a door open from the inside than the outside.

The old wife, not my mother mind you, would be sure that I would catch my death from cold after an experience like that. The cold weather causes a cold is an old wives' tale, right? Guess what? I came down with pneumonia. I didn't catch my death, but it wasn't very much fun either.

The line between truth and fact when it comes to our health can be blurry. The cold air alone did not cause me to get sick. That's a tale. But the cold air could have dried out my bronchial tubes or it could have stressed my immune system making me more susceptible to infection with viruses. We also know that cold dry weather helps to disseminate viral particles in the air. Doesn't the flu usually spread during the colder months of the year? So what is true and what isn't? That's not so easy to answer.

THE UNDERWIRE BRA

In 1992, I found a painless lump in the outer rim of my left breast. One of my first questions was "Could there be something I am doing in my day-to-day life that is causing a lump to form in my breast?" I debated between having it evaluated right away or waiting, because often it is advised to wait a couple menstrual cycles to see if it is related. My fear and need to know if it was cancer accelerated the decision for me. I decided to reach out to my colleagues for advice.

At the time, I was an internist at a medical center in San Francisco. I went to the breast care center at the university where I trained to get a biopsy. During the drive to the hospital, I had too much time alone to think. That was when the fear struck me. I had just turned 30, way too young for cancer. I just could not believe it. I started to go through my life, at first to find a cause, then just touching on all the things I still wanted to do. The list was endless.

When I got to the breast care center, I had a strange feeling. I had worked at the hospital for years, but walking in I felt like I was in a foreign country. The fear of the experience took away any familiarity I had. It helped me imagine what it might be like for my patients. The hospital was bright and clean, but that didn't dissipate any of the discomfort.

When I sat down with the doctor, it got a little worse. There was definitely a mass in my breast and I had to get tissue samples taken. Unfortunately, it didn't go too well. The doctor, who was still in his training, tried but couldn't seem to get an adequate sample, by the seventh time the needle pierced through my flesh, I felt like a pincushion. It was searing pain, like someone using a knife and going right down to my vertebrate. It was so bad, I was numb at first. Then the pain hit like a wave. When I left that day, I felt like I couldn't straighten my neck or even walk upright.

That afternoon, I went to see a silly movie to take my mind off my fear. I can't even remember the title, but I needed something to slow down the parade of dark thoughts in my head. At that time, people still weren't talking a lot about breast cancer. I think that just added to how scary a thought it was.

The movie didn't help much. When I got home, I decided to keep quiet. I didn't even share it with my family and friends. I didn't want to scare them. So I battled my fear alone, waiting for the day I would get the results.

At that time, I was in private practice. I had just finished my residency in internal medicine and was now working at Kaiser Permanente in South San Francisco. On the day I was to hear from my doctor, a patient came in with her husband. She was beside herself upset. She had just been diagnosed with a breast mass, but couldn't get a biopsy right away because of delays in scheduling. I can still picture her. She had shoulder length brown hair—a woman around my own age. She was holding her husband's hands and tears rolled down her cheeks. They both looked terrified. I tried to move the schedule up for her and to reassure that everything would be done to help her.

Once she left, I was shaken and knew I couldn't put it off any longer. I probably should have waited for my primary care doctor to call for me but I wanted to take charge. I called the pathologist directly and got the results.

They were indeterminate. I didn't know if that meant they couldn't read what they had or that they didn't have enough tissue to make a diagnosis. My heart just froze. I called again and scheduled another appointment. The second time, I knew what to expect. It was a different kind of dread going in there. I was actually focused more on the discomfort from the first visit more than the mass itself.

The second time the senior pathologist took the sample. She got it on the first try and I got my results a few days later. It was a fibroadenoma.

Fibroadenoma is generally a solid, slowly growing mass in the breast. It is usually pain free and diagnosed with a needle biopsy—or in my case—eight. Some are treated by surgically removing the lump and a small amount of normal breast tissue. It is benign.

It was great news, but you never really get over the scare. My mind went back to trying to find the cause. I had heard the claim that underwire bras can cause cancer. I remember looking into it and deciding it was a myth. I kept my bras.

Four years later, I found something suspicious in my right armpit. It just wasn't going away. My office within the Department of Health and Human Services at the time had recently awarded funding to study magnetic resonance imaging or MRI as a tool to image breasts. So I contacted the investigator for that study who was at the University of Pennsylvania. We talked and I decided to get an MRI because as a relatively young, pre-menopausal woman with dense breast tissue, I was eligible to enroll in his study. So I did.

With an IV in my arm, I was slowly wheeled on a gurney into the cold room that housed the MRI and was gently placed on the hard table. The cheap paper gown I had to wear crackled as I tried to get comfortable. It was a portent to what was coming.

When I signed the consent form, I didn't consider that I was going to be surrounded by the MRI device. I never really thought about claustrophobia before I got in there. Hearing the loud noise of the machine and feeling completely surrounded, I had to use mental imagery to get through the forty-five minutes. I pretended I was under an umbrella on the beach. I had a panic button. Boy, I was holding onto that tightly.

When they eventually changed my position, I kept thinking, "how do older people do this or anybody who has any kind of skeletal deformity?" My spine ached and the coils against my breast tissue were so uncomfortable, and a little unnerving. I felt so isolated amidst the cold metal machinery.

It hit me that I was the doctor becoming the patient. It was confusing. Part of me was intrigued. Here was a study that my office was funding. At the same time, it was my body. After the test was over, we could read the MRI results. I jumped off the table and looked at them. For a moment, it was sort of an out-of-body experience. It hit me that I was looking at the inside of my own body.

Pretty quickly, the mass was determined to be a lymph node. I felt relieved. But having a second experience like that was a good reminder that we are all human. I asked myself again, "Is there anything I've done in my life that has caused something to happen?"

I've had lots of talks with women, especially young women, who have developed breast cancer. They think, "Is it the diet? Is it not enough exercise?" "Is it due to drinking too much wine or beer?" They feel guilty because we tend to think of breast cancer as an older woman's disease.

I think that's why those thoughts come into play. What is it about the environment around us that is causing health problems? Could it be something as simple as wearing a bra? Is it due to pressure or something irritating our breast tissue? Is it my body's response to wearing the underwire?

Again, I didn't stop wearing underwire bras. I did look into it a little further this time. The first thing I did was try to uncover the source of the information. My search led to a book, *Dressed to Kill*, by Sydney Ross Singer and Soma Grismaijer. The text claimed that women wearing tight fitting bras on a daily basis are more susceptible to breast cancer. The book claimed that the bras affected the lymphatic system slowing the body's natural ability to drain toxins.

As you'd expect, people reading a serious claim like that would obviously be frightened. When we hold a book, not unlike this one, in our hands, when we see the words printed between perfectly bound hard covers, we believe them. How would we not? Weren't we taught from our first days in school that statements in books were true? Didn't our history books tell us that the War of 1812 was fought in 1812 or that Christopher Columbus discovered America?

Unfortunately, as we eventually come to find out, some things that are printed may not be true. Yet, it is still hard to not believe in them. When I dug deeper, I found that the American Cancer Society has determined that there is no link between bras and cancer. Some scientists have reviewed the couple's findings and found insufficient evidence to support it. They question the control of the authors' research, claiming other risk factors for breast cancer were not considered. You have to ask yourself what was the reason for them to take this stand and defend it.

After my research, I decided there was not enough evidence to support the myth that my underwire bra was causing cancer. It got me thinking, what other myths are out there? And what might they be doing to our health?

MAMMOGRAPHY

In November 2009, an explosive debate erupted in the world of medicine. I'm not talking about health care reform, although what I am referring to affect the debate. The issue revolved around mammograms not saving lives.

In the fall of 2009, the U.S. Preventive Services Task Force (USPSTF), an independent panel of scientists, epidemiologists and doctors, released new guidelines for woman concerning breast health. They stated that women in their 40s should stop having routine mammograms. For women over fifty, they recommended cutting back to one exam every other year. The report claimed that the potential harm of having annual exams outweighed their benefit. Additionally, they recommended against self-exams and found insufficient evidence to recommend that doctors do breast exams. One caveat was that women should consider early screenings if they had risk factors for breast cancer or relatives with the disease.

The findings could not have come at a more charged time. The country was enmeshed in a health care reform debate and people were worried about the possibility of rationing care. On top of that, reaction to the findings was polarized. Some groups lauded the findings. Part of the task force's reasoning was that the test produced high false-positive results especially in the younger age groups. They believed that this would lead to increased patient anxiety and unnecessary further testing that could be harmful. They also cited the risk of increased radiation exposure from the tests.

The Task Force's findings were in part based on findings of over 40 studies, including a British study that involved over 160,000 women and data collected from 600,000 American women. The task force also commissioned their own modeling study that involved six separate teams of researchers.

They acknowledged that annual mammograms for women over forty reduced the mortality rate by 15 percent. What they concluded, though, was that of 1000 women screened starting at forty; only two to four would get a diagnosis of breast cancer. At the same time, they found that 470 women would get a false-positive result. Interestingly, they even compared conventional mammography to other studies including digital mammography that uses the same type of silicon chips that are found in the Hubble telescope which converts light into an image. They found no additional benefit overall for women even with these other tests. Even NASA technology did not confer an advantage.

The reaction to this news intensified when the Secretary of the Department of Health and Human Services at that time, Kathleen Sebelius, issued a statement soon after the release of the report suggesting women continue to get regular mammograms starting at forty. Her response fueled a backlash from opponents of health care reform. They stated that it was an example of what would happen if the government controlled healthcare and that this issue was driven by economic concerns on the backs or "chests" of women.

It is no wonder that these findings elicited a dramatic response. Look around. Everything has been "pinkized." At the time of the findings, even National Football League players were wearing pink gloves and pink shoes as a sign of solidarity toward the fight against breast cancer. In October 2008, I returned from Panama were everything was draped in pink, including parts of the airport to show support for breast cancer awareness. Advocates and health professionals had worked tirelessly to educate the public that they needed to get breast exams and to become familiar with their breasts in order to find masses when they were small. Early detection could save lives was drilled into our minds.

I was not surprised by the report nor the public outcry and the Administration's response. It was 1997 all over again. At that time, I was invited to serve on a high level work group that the DHHS formed in response to the National Cancer Institute's Consensus Conference statements about breast cancer screenings which were remarkably similar to the 2009 guidelines. In 1997, breast cancer awareness was gaining momentum. President Clinton was a strong advocate since his mother died from the disease and the First Lady, Hillary Rodham Clinton, traveled the country highlighting Medicare's coverage for mammograms. I had even been in Rome to speak at the first Susan G. Komen Race for the Cure which took place around the Coliseum and the Forum. Not only the United States but also the world was interested in breast cancer as large numbers of women with the disease began to speak up and demand more action to prevent, diagnose and treat it.

In 1997, we were ushered into the conference room of the Secretary's office and sat at a long beautiful wooden table. Representatives from the National Cancer Institute, the Office of Women's Health and Public Affairs participated. Legislative Affairs and Media Relations professionals were there too. It was an extremely tense meeting. We realized then we were walking on a political landmine.

Congress planned to hold hearings on the issue. As it turned out, the Senate would unanimously pass a nonbinding resolution to strongly urge screenings for this 40+ age group—a recommendation that the National Cancer Institute adopted to no surprise.

During the meeting, we discussed the quality of data presented and the ramifications of policy. Even then, we knew that the mammogram was an old test—over forty years old. We needed to offer women something better, but it wasn't there. Our work group was very concerned about the false negatives in this age range since we knew that breast cancer can be especially aggressive in younger women. So we suggested that the testing be annually just in case a mass was missed, hoping that by the following year, it might be detected and treated.

The 2009 findings just highlighted our 1997 concerns even more. The obvious answer to these findings is that we need better testing. Can you imagine if men had to get the same test on their testicles? Not only would the test have been revamped to be less painful long ago, but if results like these showed up, a new test would be demanded and found. As we enter the world of personalized medicine, hopefully, we will develop biomarkers which will help us to detect masses early and also to find the ones that can actually cause invasive disease.

My recommendation to women in this age group is to continue to get mammograms annually beginning at forty. I find the claim of protecting women from the anxiety of false-positives to be insulting and patronizing. As for the issue of radiation exposure, it is not enough to warrant not getting them done—the amount in a standard mammogram is 13 rems which are about the same as a person would naturally absorb from the environment in three months.

Women have been getting the test for decades and through the Mammography Quality Screening Act, imaging centers now need to be certified and found to conduct safe and reliable exams. The challenge is to ensure that radiologists are well trained to detect small masses and that the results are reported timely and accurately.

As for breast self exams, it is an opportunity for women to learn more about their bodies. Breast tissue is normally "lumpy and bumpy." By doing it regularly, perhaps every couple of months, women will grow more comfortable and know what feels normal for them. I cannot stress how important it is if you find a lump to get it evaluated by your doctor. It is also recommended to get your mammogram about a week after your menstrual period. Your breasts are very sensitive to the estrogen and progesterone levels in your body and the levels are the lowest then—

this may make the test more comfortable for you as well. And remember to not wear deodorants which can cause irregular spots to appear on your mammogram—I learned that lesson the hard way!

These findings should be a calling card for other diseases that are often under or misdiagnosed in women, such as heart disease. Minimally invasive and more sensitive tests are needed. Saying don't get screened is not a responsible option. Just because a test may not prove a diagnosis, does not mean that the disease does not exist.

Ideally, this situation could have been seen as a learning opportunity. Time should have been taken and results discussed on how to communicate the information before such inflammatory results were shared. Instead, an environment of fear and confusion was created. Although the Secretary said that the recommendations and guidelines were not mandates which needed to be followed, the damage had been done. The strength of the Task Force was diminished by the public outcry and subsequent statements and actions taken by the Administration and Congress.

The U.S. Preventive Services Task Force was doing their best job to evaluate the data that is in existence. They are not driven by economic concerns. They also had the challenging task to conduct statistical evaluation of studies that focus on the data from a large population perspective. So if only one woman would be saved out of a group of 1900 women screened, we all want to be that one woman. It is human nature and we need to acknowledge that. Until society deems it impossible to save one life because of economic constraints, this type of policy decision cannot be made.

The fallout from this communication debacle resulted in Congress passing legislation to require health insurance companies to provide free mammograms for women, especially for women forty and older, and additional preventive services to women such as screenings for other cancers, heart disease and diabetes as well as post-partum depression and domestic violence.

Many suggested that the Task Force had yielded too much power and influence on health policy, and that they conducted their meetings behind closed doors without public discourse or oversight. Mammography coverage may have been the final straw for legislators who needed to respond to their constituents who were already afraid that they would lose or not receive health insurance benefits.

The mammography controversy demonstrated the complexity of making policy decisions in the midst of powerful psycho-social and political forces shaping the environment. No decision can be solely based on scientific findings though they should guide the process. Good common sense is the compass, the tool to navigate the universe of colliding worlds.

DEODORANTS

Here is another rumor that generates fear. Antiperspirants used by women cause cancer. The concept is similar to the underwire bra. It claims that the chemicals in the antiperspirant affect the lymph nodes' ability to purge harmful chemicals.

As it did with the underwire bra scare, the scientific community does not support this claim. Much like the reaction to the book *Dressed to Kill*, health organizations had to respond to the rumor because enough people took it to heart and were afraid.

A study done addressing the link between antiperspirants and cancer attempted to provide evidence that there was no connection between usage and breast cancer. They investigated a "possible relationship between use of products applied for underarm perspiration and the risk for breast cancer in women aged 20-74." Their findings found no significant link. To their knowledge, this study was the only "epidemiologic evidence" relating to the rumored link.

When trying to uncover the facts, often different studies will come to different conclusions. Sometimes when you review literature, you'll find views that are polar opposites. It adds to the challenge of uncovering the truth.

There are steps you can take to help educate yourself. You can look at the journal to see if they publish peer-reviewed articles. Do the researchers have any apparent bias? Look at the study's parameters. Does the sample size seem representative of the population? Is the study funded by industry? Does it look as if the study was well designed? After that, talk to your doctor. Find a doctor that is up-to-date on the literature and can share the findings with you in a balanced manner.

To add to the complication, the Internet is a great source that you should use carefully. Discussion groups are good group therapy, but the medical advice dispensed there should not be considered 100 percent factual. When looking at health information online, consider what site you are looking at and who funds it. Because it is on the computer screen does not mean it is the voice of truth.

TAMPONS

One of the most prevalent rumors relating to women's health is the danger of tampons. Tens of millions of women in this country use tampons. Every woman is warned not to leave them in too long or not to use high-absorbing brands. As much fear and misunderstanding shadow the product as does the female menstrual cycle itself.

During my work with NASA, the menstrual cycle was an interesting topic. Women on Earth cycle along with the moon. What would our cycle be if we lived on the moon, then? Would we align ourselves back to the movement of the Earth? What happens when we are orbiting the Earth every 90 minutes? Would cycles be impacted if we landed on Mars and the days are longer?

Other concerns came up as well. What about retrograde flow or having menstrual blood flow backwards into the fallopian tubes and out into the abdomen. Gravity causes everything to flow down on Earth, but what happens without gravity while in space? It was feared that the lack of gravity pushing menstrual fluid out could lead to endometriosis in female astronauts. Studies of pilots have shown it doesn't, but it is still a topic of conversation.

Everything is a little harder to do in space, whether it is eating, sleeping, or hygiene. But a menstrual period is not an abnormality. I consider it a vital sign. When women are too thin or too stressed, their menstrual cycles are altered and menses or periods may stop all together.

It is no wonder rumors have revolved around tampons. The first such rumor to discuss is that tampons cause cancer. This came about when it was reported that harmful toxins were used in the process to manufacture the product. One of the most hazardous toxins is dioxin. Some of the rumors also included asbestos. A third arm of the story is that the rayon in tampons causes toxic shock syndrome.

As for dioxins, they are a byproduct of the process that makes rayon and trace amounts can be found in the fiber afterwards. They have been found to be a carcinogen. Dioxins have also been linked to other serious illnesses, including endometriosis.

Researchers examined whether dioxins in tampons increased the risk of women developing endometriosis. They found that the amount of exposure to the toxins through tampons amounted to "six orders of magnitude lower than estimated daily food exposure levels to these contaminants." They also found that there is inconsistent evidence pointing to environmental exposure to dioxins causing endometriosis.

Asbestos claims are less founded. Some rumors stated that tampon companies purposely included asbestos in tampons to promote menstrual bleeding, thus increasing the demand for their product. In response, the FDA claimed that no tampons sold in the US contain asbestos as an ingredient.

The rumors swirling around tampons made it all the way to Congress. In 1997, I went up to Capitol Hill with my colleagues from the Office on Women's Health to talk to members of the Congressional Caucus on Women's Issues about dioxin in tampons. Their constituents were upset that their health could be hurt by using tampons and wanted reassurance that they were safe. It was a cordial meeting, but we did not have lots of data to share at that time.

Congresswoman Carolyn Maloney introduced legislation, "The Robin Danielson Act," that tasked the National Institutes of Health to uncover the amount of dioxins, as well as any additive that could put a woman's health at risk, in tampons. It also called on the Centers for Disease Control and Prevention (CDC) to report back on the prevalence of toxic shock syndrome. According to her press release, "the bill is named for a woman who died from the illness."

This was not Representative Maloney's first bill concerning tampon safety. She also introduced "The Tampon Safety and Research Act of 1997," after our meeting, and "The Robin Danielson Act" in 2005, 2003 and 1999.

We definitely wanted to expand the research. No matter what, women are still going to use tampons and needed answers. Many studies have focused on superabsorbent tampons and their link to toxic shock syndrome.

In 2005, a study cited congressional interest as a reason to examine the amount of dioxin and furan in tampons. Tampon samples were analyzed. The findings stated that levels of dioxins and furans were below the limit of detection. So, according to the research, it does not seem that dioxins in tampons cause endometriosis or cancer. But what about toxic shock syndrome? Could that part of the rumor be true?

People should be aware of the risk of tampon use and toxic shock syndrome. I remember seeing a woman in the ER at Bellevue Hospital in New York City who had all the signs and symptoms of this disease. She came to the ER because she was concerned that the skin on her palms was shedding and her face was bright red. While talking to her, she admitted that she would keep tampons in for over 24 hours. Shortly afterwards, my roommate was using a contraceptive sponge and couldn't get it out. She went into the ER to get it extracted because she was worried about toxic shock syndrome. That was in the mid 1980s and frightening stories about tampons and contraceptive sponges causing toxic shock syndrome circulated widely in the media.

Toxic shock syndrome is a real medical condition caused by bacteria. It has been linked to leaving a tampon in for longer than is recommended and using high-absorbing tampons made of rayon. According to the FDA, about half of the cases can be tied back to tampon use. Interestingly, men, children and non-menstruating women can also develop toxic shock syndrome. To put the problem into perspective, in 1980, 814 cases were reported. In 1997, that number was five. Creative communication strategies to educate the public on the need to frequently change tampons worked.

How I see it, tampons are a great example of facing a myth head on and digging deep enough to find the kernel of truth. It also touched on how politics and the public can influence health discussions whether it starts in the press or a constituent's phone call to her congresswoman.

HAIR DYES

I once gave a speech to a number of military doctors in San Antonio, Texas. It was a Sunday morning and I was talking about the development of novel technologies for imaging breast tissue. I discussed some of the latest devices that were coming out of the CIA, NASA, and the Department of Defense. For example, I discussed the CIA use of neural networks in computer imagery to pinpoint missile strikes in the first Gulf War. Could this same technology be used to pinpoint cancer cells in breast tissue?

At the end of my talk, a physician in the back row, an older gentleman, raised his hand.

"I may have more gray hair than you, so I warn you to be careful about these technologies," he said. "They need to be tested."

I was amused by his comment. He equated gray hair with knowledge, and I had just had my hair highlighted the day before to camouflage some hypo-pigmented strands. So I said, tongue in cheek, "Sir, we have technologies to take care of your gray hair." The generals in the front row applauded and laughed.

His statement covered a couple of biases, including gender and age. He was reminding me that in his day, a lot of technologies that were supposed to be great never did pan out. In his patronizing style, he voiced that opinion. I assured him that all these tools needed to be evaluated for safety and efficacy, not to mention the cost of doing them on a large scale first.

In his way, he was right. We need to be careful of what we read and where it appears; and we should look to scientific studies to find the truth. At times, I've seen patients bring in articles from the *National Enquirer* or from a website that is designed to sell a product or promote an ideology, thinking the medical claims made were valid. It is false advertising that can do much harm.

The conversation also got me thinking about hair dye and the rumor that it causes cancer. In the early nineties, the International Agency for Research on Cancer (IARC), the body that classifies carcinogens, examined hair dye for just that reason. Their classifications range from known human carcinogens to probably not carcinogenic. After reviewing the data, the IARC determined there was not enough evidence to classify hair dye as a carcinogen.

Since then, more studies have been conducted but little to no evidence has been found to implicate hair dye as a major factor in cancer development. One study specifically examined hair product usage and the risk of breast cancer and found that neither hair coloring nor hair spray increases breast cancer risk. For those of us who like to change our looks now and then this is reassuring news.

HEART DISEASE

Women and heart disease is an issue that now raises much passion. It was not always the case. I often think back to a lecture I attended in the 1990s. Dr. Bernadine Healy was the speaker. She was the first woman to be named Director of the National Institutes of Health and a giant in the field of women's health. She told us a story about a conference on heart disease that advertised to women. As she drove up to the conference site hosting the event, she saw a line of cars waiting to get in. More women than she could have imagined, all ready to listen and be educated. When she got inside, she found out the title of the session. It was "How do women help their men with heart disease." Perhaps, a shocking title to us now, but not at that time.

That story personifies what I hear all the time. Some still believe the myth that women do not develop heart disease. When I was a medical student at New York University in the late 1980s, I saw a woman in her fifties who only spoke Spanish. The resident who was teaching me translated and told me that the patient was complaining of shoulder pain and nausea. Since she also appeared anxious and breathing very quickly, my resident ordered a "white milkshake"—a concoction of Valium and Mylanta to calm her down. For the six hours that she was allowed to stay—the magical number for ER visits, she slept. Anyone given 10 mg of Valium would do the same. She was then discharged to home and told to go to her doctor to follow-up on the bursitis in her shoulder and her indigestion. An hour later, she came back in full cardiac arrest. She had been having a myocardial infarction or a heart attack while in the ER. It was a misdiagnosis. A simple EKG was never done during her first visit.

Women are often described as having "atypical" symptoms for heart disease such as jaw pain, nausea, shoulder pain or shortness of breath, but these are actually "typical" for women. I learned an important lesson that day which influenced how I would practice medicine and teach my medical students and interns. I admitted many women with these symptoms when I was a resident in internal medicine at the University of California, San Francisco and, sure enough, they were having heart attacks.

We know that women have been under-diagnosed. That is why the National Heart, Lung, and Blood Institute launched the Red Dress campaign and American Heart Association launched the Go Red campaign to expand awareness of heart disease in women. Both programs target women of all ages.

In my opinion, the claim that only men suffer from cardiovascular heart disease is a dangerous myth. Not just that, it is a deadly old wives' tale that could lead to heartbreak, literally.

ABORTION

Serving as the medical advisor for women's health during both a conservative administration and a more liberal one, I have seen first hand how politics can influence the birth and life of a myth. Immediately, my mind turns to abortion. There are few topics as politicized. So, it would be interesting to look at the myth that abortions increase the risk of cancer.

Some studies have found that women's hormones may increase the risk of getting some types of breast cancer. The levels of hormones such as estrogen, prolactin and progesterone are significantly elevated during pregnancy. Since abortion affects the body's natural cycle guiding these levels, it is not surprising that a link between abortion and cancer arises.

In 1996, researchers examined data from reports published on breast health to determine if there was a link between abortion and breast cancer. In all, they analyzed 28 published reports to determine the odds ratio of developing cancer after an abortion. Although very low, they concluded that abortion could be considered a significant independent risk factor. They approximated thousands of additional cases per year attributed to abortions.

On the contrary, a Danish study found differently. According to the American Cancer Society, this study is considered the most reliable because of that nation's impressive medical records keeping. All women born over a 40 year period, over a million, registered with both the National Registry of Induced Abortion and the Cancer Registry. Based on their extensive database, researchers came to the conclusion that abortions do not increase a woman's risk of cancer.

In 2003, some of the world's leading doctors specializing in breast cancer diagnosis and treatment came together for a National Cancer Institute symposium. Although they found that there is some increased risk of developing breast cancer shortly after delivering a full term baby, it was decided that there was no link to cancer and abortion.

It makes you wonder how much the political charge of an issue like abortion affects the science of medical studies. I remember when I started at the Office of Women's Health within the Department Health and Human Services having to immediately wrestle with this issue. In 1994, an article just published by the National Cancer Institute linked abortion and breast cancer. An advocacy group quickly placed an ad in the Metro stations in response to this article. It was a picture of a young woman cupping her breast protectively. The caption read, "Women who choose abortion suffer more and deadlier breast cancer." According to transcripts from a legal case based in Philadelphia, Dr. Philip Lee, the Assistant Secretary of Health and Human Services at the time, sent a letter to the Washington Metropolitan Area Transit Authority calling the ads "misleading, unduly alarming, and does not accurately reflect the weight of scientific literature." He added that, in his opinion, the study had weak methodology and that he knew of no scientific basis for correlating abortion with "deadlier" breast cancer.

The ads were pulled quickly because of the general reaction. I remember taking press calls on the issue. We looked into it, reviewed the data and refuted it. Unfortunately, in some ways, it was too late to negate the impact.

Sometimes just being accused can derail a position or even a career. It makes me think about the man who was accused of the Olympic bombings in Atlanta, Eric Robert Rudolph. His life was never the same after that accusation even though he was innocent.

Once again, if it is a myth, is it believable by being backed up by an ounce of science? For example, we know that hormones affect breast cancer development. But there is not enough science to make outrageous claims like the ad from the Metro. Such claims cause fear, and I don't want women to be frightened or made to feel guilty if they do develop breast cancer.

*   *   *

Myths can evolve from stories that people tell, passed down from generation to generation. They can also be born of real data. When subsequent data refutes it, a kernel of the original story remains, growing roots on its own. Myths also originate from fear. People are often not comfortable living with the unknown. So we may fill in the doubt and fear with stories.

It is the science of medicine that extracts the truth from the myth. Yet, we might not be able to prove all the points without a shadow of doubt. That is where the art of medicine comes in to play. Doctors need to take in the full picture of their patients, and patients need to take in a full picture of their lives.

In 2005, I was in a shop in Beijing, China that had a table full of lingerie, actually lovely items for only a dollar a piece. The woman working behind the table told me I was too big for her bras, but I didn't believe her since I had never been told that line before. So I found the size that related to my size back home and bought a number of them. It was hard to turn away from such a great sale price. Although attractive, I don't think they were designed with the American body in mind. They weren't all that comfortable.

A year later, I received an early morning call from the George Washington University Breast Health Center that my mammogram now showed micro-calcifications in my right breast. Regardless of my experience as a doctor, or the research I had done when I had my scares years before, the first thought that popped into my mind was, "Is it the bra again?"

I made an appointment to be seen that afternoon. I sat in the waiting room at the hospital, sweating through my cloth gown this time even though the air conditioning was on full blast. I decided that if the reading was again abnormal, I was still going on a hiking trip in France that I had planned to start the next day. It was my way to take control of frightening situation. I was experiencing all the feelings of dread, fear and anxiety that I had with prior visits to deal with my breasts.

I always joked with my sisters that I must have inherited my dad's genes for breast size while my two sisters had my mom's genes since the women in my family were quite buxom. I could always wear a sports bra and jog miles without a problem. Yet, I was the one having to frequently face breast health issues.

I repeated the mammogram with more views of my breasts and it was decided that the abnormality seen on the first one may have been due to the deodorant that I did not fully wash off before the test. In fact, you are told to make sure your skin is totally clean and free of any products before the test. The irony didn't pass me by. My deodorant caused the "fear" of cancer. It makes it easy to see how there has to be some element of truth to these rumors or they wouldn't spread.

Myths are insidious things. Like weeds, their roots dig deep and hold tight. To complicate the issue, politics and gender can get into the game, making it even harder to ferret out the truth. All you can do is ask your doctor, do some research especially using government websites and publications and, in the end, do what you think is right.

After that mammogram, I did discard those bras from China. Maybe I did that because the science could not completely weed out the myth rooted in my traumatized memory. Maybe they were just really uncomfortable. Or maybe it was because I hope someday to go to space and there is no sag in zero-g. Does the reason matter? It does show that no matter how educated you are, or how wise, or how much gray hair you have, myths are easy to believe and worth the time to investigate.

Stellar Questions:

If you sit too close to the television, will you go blind?

If this one was true, I would need strong glasses. I have vivid memories of sitting with my nose almost touching the screen while we watched the Apollo mission. It might have been the excitement of the times or how grainy the picture was, but most of the world was probably sitting that close.

The myth may have some truth in the past. It probably came from the fact that early televisions emitted higher amounts of radiation that could have caused vision issues. Modern television sets don't appear to have that problem. A study found heredity to be the most important risk factor of children developing myopia or near-sightedness. Sitting too close to a television set was not listed as a risk factor.

Do pesticides have an ill effect on women's health?

I love to garden. I'm very protective of every square inch of my lawn. I live in the Washington, D.C. where open space is pretty valuable. Sometimes I use pesticides on my lawn, but I don't like doing that very often. I always wash my hands afterwards and wear closed toe shoes. The most important thing is that I follow the directions on the product.

Being around my plants is relaxing. It is my oasis. But to have an oasis, I was concerned that I have used chemicals. Unfortunately, the Department of Health and Human Services thinks this one is true. It seems pretty straightforward. Pesticides are made to kill unwanted living organisms. The U.S. National Safety Council's website lists products registered with the Environmental Protection Agency (EPA). It recommends that you carefully follow product instructions and use pesticides in a well-ventilated place. Researches did a review of the data and found it "suggestive of increased risks of fetal deaths associated with pesticides in general."

It seems obvious, but wear gloves and protective clothing too. The less you're exposed the better.

Can I eat sushi if I'm pregnant?

This one makes me think back to my residency in San Francisco, a city filled with great Japanese restaurants. At the time, I was training in an infectious disease clinic. I saw many exotic diseases in that clinic. Before that rotation, I loved to eat sushi. I always stuck to the California rolls. The one time I had raw fish, I felt ill afterwards. I sat up all night wondering what parasite I absorbed into my body.

While working in the clinic, I was asked if pregnant women should avoid sushi. You'll get different answers to this one depending on whom you ask. Obstetricians in the United States may say "yes." Doctors in Japan may say "no." So what is the truth?

There are two parts to the question to be concerned about—food borne illness and mercury exposure. I once saw a patient at San Francisco General Hospital who had anisakiasis from consuming raw fish infected with anisakidae—parasites. Soon after ingesting the parasite, severe pain, nausea and vomiting starts. If the anisakidae reach the bowel, more serious problems arise, usually an infection that shows itself a week or two later. On top of that, the parasite releases a biochemical compound that can cause an allergic response in some people.

If that's not enough, you could get other bacterial infections such as salmonella. So at the very least, some caution should be given to eating raw fish while pregnant or any time for that matter. Make sure that the restaurants are serving fresh fish, the sushi bars are clean and there are no health violations.

Mercury levels in fish have been rising. Mercury is not good for you. It can cause neurological damage. According to the FDA, tuna isn't the biggest culprit. That title goes to the tilefish in the Gulf of Mexico, followed by swordfish, shark and king mackerel. The larger fish has more mercury. The American Pregnancy Association recommends no more than 12 ounces of low mercury containing fish a week and 18 ounces a month for high mercury containing fish.

Will I lose my memory when I get older?

Evidence seems to show that age related memory loss is not as inevitable and irreversible as it once was believed to be. No longer is it universally believed that memory loss is caused by the death of neurons in the brain as we age. Additionally, there are studies that show the connections between neurons may be damaged.

Alzheimer's disease is the one of the most notorious and irreversible brain conditions plaguing our aging population. It is the most common cause of dementia in the elderly and, according to the Alzheimer's Research and Prevention Foundation, is suffered by 5.3 million Americans. Right now there is no "magic bullet" treatment for the disease. Some drugs help slow the progress of the disease, but nothing has been able to reverse the progression of the illness.

According to the National Institute on Aging, research suggests that exercise and a healthy diet can help. Specifically, older people with higher levels of exercise are at a lower risk of suffering dementia. In

2005, a study in Nature Neuroscience also claimed that memory loss in senior citizens may be related to an inability to filter out distractions. In their study, they found younger people were able to suppress brain activity that did not have to do with memory. Older adults were less able to do that.

I believe that keeping the mind active is the most important thing we can do as we age. I encouraged my father to take a summer class at the local college by saying I would take one at the same time. We had a lot of enjoyment driving together and talking about what we learned afterwards. Besides taking classes, do crosswords puzzles or read regularly. And don't forget to exercise—dance around the house—anything to keep your mind active. As we have learned from research conducted in space, there is neuronal plasticity. Neurons can rewire in response to new stimulus. It is never too late to learn a new language or a dance step.

Can blueberries control diabetes?

It's no wonder blueberries are thought to be a super food. Their health benefits can be traced back to well before any settlers set foot on to North America. The Native Americans used blueberries, as well as the leaves and roots of the plant, as medicine. Even further back, the berries are also found in Russian folk medicine.

Blueberries contain vitamins, phenolics and anthocyanins which can act as antioxidants or molecules that help prevent the production of cell damaging free radicals. Anthocyanins may also help fight dementia as we age as well. A recent study showed that blueberries may in fact be beneficial to diabetics. Researchers found that the berry contains insulin-like properties and protects against glucose toxicity.

The National Cancer Institute suggests eating five or more servings of fruit and vegetables each day. They specifically suggest blue and purple fruits, including blueberries. Steven Pratt, M.D., the author of *Super Foods Rx: Fourteen Foods to Change Your Life*, calls them "brain berries" Somehow, my parents must have known that because I was raised on blueberries. We had them every morning with our cereal before we left for school.

Can chicken soup treat a cold?

Much like blueberries, I was raised on chicken soup. It was a cultural practice. We called it "Jewish penicillin." The tradition of using it as the best medicine for a cold was passed down through generations. On top of that, it was featured in religious meals such as the Sabbath dinner.

Not surprisingly, there is an element of truth to chicken soup's reputation as a wonder drug. According to researchers, chicken soup has been found to have "beneficial medicinal activity." They found that the soup might have an anti-inflammatory effect which helps upper respiratory tract infections. Stephen Rennard, M.D., tested his wife's chicken soup in a lab. They found that it affected white blood cells and decreased the symptoms related to the common cold. The beneficial effect was found in all the ingredients in the soup, but the chicken did not have anti-inflammatory activity. Furthermore, store-bought soups performed less reliably.

In this case, the old wives' tale has been proven more accurate than most. Previously, we knew that the steam can help congestion, the broth and electrolytes can keep you hydrated and soup is good for diarrhea. A pot of homemade chicken soup is worth a pound of cure.

Do antibiotics decrease the effectiveness of oral contraceptives?

This can be true. I once saw a patient at a Kaiser Urgent Care Center who was concerned because she hadn't had her period. I started asking her questions regarding her sexual activity and contraceptive use and whether she had any recent infections. She said that she used birth control pills because she was sexually active and was also on antibiotics for an upper respiratory infection. I did a pregnancy test and it came back positive. She was in shock.

Historically, Rifampicin and Griseofulvin are known to alter the effectiveness of oral contraception. Rifampicin was originally used along with other drugs to treat tuberculosis. Griseofulvin is used to treat fungal infections. Many studies differ; however, when looking at broad-spectrum antibiotics. So, to be safe, have back up contraception when you are using antibiotics.

Can brushing my teeth decrease my risk of having a heart attack?

There is definitely truth to this. Dental health professionals have long believed that the mouth plays an important role in overall wellness. A scientist from the University of Buffalo, Oelisoa Andriankaja, identified two bacteria found in the mouth *Tannerella forsynthesis* and *Prevotella intermedia* in patients who had suffered heart attacks. The researchers caution that it is not necessarily what type of bacteria, but simply the amount of bacteria that is entering the blood through poor dental health.

The idea is that poor dental health can lead to bleeding gums. The open wounds then let bacteria into the blood stream which activates the immune system and the development of vascular plaque.

Interestingly, antibodies to Chlamydia have been found in patients with heart disease. *Chlamydia pneumoniae* is a common cause of respiratory disease. It is believed to cause 10 percent of community-acquired pneumonia and five percent of pharyngitis, bronchitis and sinusitis.

The theory is that the immune system's response to invading bacteria can lead to the build up of plaque in blood vessels, much like it leads to plaque on teeth. A study examining the presence of bacterial proteins in atherosclerotic plaque found 50 different species. This may show that it is the plethora of infection that increases risk as opposed to a single pathogen.

Does an apple a day can keep the doctor away?

Apples have played an important part in the history of civilization as shared through many stories. Eve took a bite of the forbidden fruit and had to leave Paradise. Paris gave the golden apple to Aphrodite, thus starting the Trojan War. And the apple fell on Sir Isaac Newton's head, introducing gravity.

It's no wonder this one statement is deeply rooted in our culture. Apple skin contains flavonoids. In plants, flavonoids help provide color and protection from insects. For humans, they are an antioxidant which can help repair cell damage from free oxygen radicals and may help prevent diseases.

So eat an apple a day. It can't hurt. But don't keep the doctor too far away.

Can bed rest help to decrease back pain?

It used to be that bed rest was considered the starting point for recovery. Even when I was in medical school, we were taught that rest helped decompress pressure on the body. Times have changed. Now, it is hospital policy for staff to get patients up and walking soon after surgery even after major procedures.

Now we understand that the human body is designed for movement. The space program has taught us a bit about this. We've seen that in space, astronauts can experience back pain as the ligaments and discs stretch due to the lack of gravity and shifting of body fluid. They even get taller while floating around in the microgravity environment of space. Some return to Earth with back problems from these changes. Physical therapy helps to decrease pain and increase mobility for the astronaut corps as well.

It is useful in some circumstances to take it easy in the short term. But after that, movement improves circulation and coordination. Bodies lose calcium when lying in bed for too long. Calcium is leached from the bones, possibly weakening them, and can deposit in joints or be lost in the urine or stool. We need movement to stay healthy and strong.

CHAPTER THREE
WOMB ON THE MOON
—A Galactic View of Women's Health

"Life without sex might be safer but it would be unbearably dull. It is the sex instinct which makes women seem beautiful, which they are once in a blue moon, and men seem wise and brave, which they never are at all. Throttle it, denaturalize it, take it away, and human existence would be reduced to the prosaic, laborious, bore some imbecile level of life in an anthill."

—H. L. Mencken

A woman will set foot on the moon. What will she be known for? Will it be her accomplishments as an astronaut or for being the first woman on the moon? Will it be a small step for a woman, but a giant leap for womankind? I hope that we will have made enough social progress by then so that it will be for all of humankind. But, we have many miles to go on this journey before we can say for certain that we will accept this universal concept. We can look at women's health as the reflection of these attitudes and beliefs.

From our country's polarizing views of sex to the short sighted "bikini medicine" of the mid 20th century, women's health has been politicized. It is important for us to understand why it has happened and explore a little deeper before making what could be life or death medical decisions. From my time working with NASA, I found space to be the perfect frontier to put this issue into perspective.

Ever since I was a little girl I couldn't decide whether to be a doctor or an explorer. I can still remember the excitement I had in the 1960s, boarding an airplane to go to New York City, wearing my white gloves and best dress. My twin brother, wearing a suit with a little bow tie that day, joined me on my adventure to the sky. We were so excited that we could barely sit in our seats when the stewardess, as she was called back then, gave us our wings to pin on our clothes. We were now official pilots on a trip to the clouds.

When our dinner was served, I was amazed. I still remember the chicken and peas on the tray. Even though it was probably just a TV dinner that we loved to eat in the 1960s, I could not believe that I was eating something hot and familiar at 30,000 feet above the Earth. There was something special about being served food in the air.

We flew back home on July 4, 1969. As we took off, I saw fireworks blending in with the stars in the sky. I felt like I was heading to the moon! A line from the song, Best That You Can Do, from the movie Arthur— "When you get caught between the moon and New York City" still plays in my head when I think about that trip. Those moments changed my life. You have to understand, in a few weeks, a man would walk on the moon.

I will never forget July 20, 1969—the day that we walked on the moon! My family went to dinner at the Yum Yum Tree, a huge Polynesian buffet restaurant in Denver, Colorado. During dinner among the fake palm trees and bamboo plants, an announcement was made that the Eagle, the vehicle carrying our astronauts to the moon, was about to land. Everyone in the restaurant ate quickly and we all rushed home. I sat inches away from our old black and white television wanting to capture every second of the grainy pictures from a world that seemed so far away yet so close to my heart.

I held my breath when Neil Armstrong took that first step. I told my parents that I wanted to go to the moon too. I remember looking at the moon that night from my bedroom window and wishing that one day, we would go back and forth to the moon in planes just like my flight to New York City a few weeks before. That was a flight that I definitely wanted to be on.

I was in grade school then and during the days and months following the first lunar landing, the teacher would bring a television into the classroom. We'd all watch the Apollo astronauts—transfixed to their every movement that they made on the lunar surface. We were mesmerized by their kangaroo hops. It became a part of our education. It was the way I grew up.

From then on, I often sat with my parents in our house in Colorado, looking at the moon and wanting to be closer to it. Thankfully, they didn't tell me that women weren't allowed in the space program. It would not be until 1983 when Sally Ride finally traveled to space. They knew how much I wanted to see what was up there.

As I grew older and got interested in medicine, I began to wonder how space travel could be important when we faced such serious health needs on Earth. I wrote a long letter in my 12-year-old hand to President Nixon, asking why we funded space travel when what we really needed was a cure for cancer. I can remember getting a reply in an envelope labeled simply "The White House," without a street address, but the letter didn't answer my question. It was just an auto-pen signed picture of Richard Nixon and a short note thanking me for the correspondence of our young constituents.

For several years I lost interest in being an astronaut in favor of pursuing medicine. That changed when I attended Barnard College and took an astronomy class with Dr. Robert Jastrow. It was an evening class at Columbia University. He would talk about the birth and death of stars and the influence of the moon on our planet.

Even though it was one of my elective classes, I absolutely loved going to it. Dr. Jastrow was a charismatic individual. One of his offices was a NASA office, above of all places Tom's Restaurant, the one in the scene from the Seinfeld television show on Broadway near Columbia University. I would go over and drop off my papers there. Seeing the NASA logo on the door always took my breath away.

This professor awakened all my former awe of the heavens, and I couldn't wait to get back to class each night. It was in his class that I reaffirmed my belief that humans are made from the same celestial dust that is in space, and my childhood drive to go to the stars was rekindled. Fifteen years later, I was able to join NASA as a doctor and medical advisor.

Twice now during my work with NASA, I've been in the running to become an astronaut, and I still have that hunger to be part of a program that ventures to new worlds. Being involved with space exploration has allowed me to stretch my mind to what's possible. For someone who loves medicine and science, it is simply the ultimate thrill.

As I get older, if I were to become an astronaut, I'd probably be the one doing studies on hot flashes in space, but for now I'm content to be part of the terrestrial or Earth-based team that studies medicine and space travel, especially the areas that have to do with women's health. The extreme environment of space flight allows us to see women's health in a stark light, and helps us to focus on what's really important to know and to study. It also teaches us possible approaches to the most common health issues we face on Earth.

As a doctor, I am endlessly fascinated by the effects of space travel on the human body. Let me give you an example. We now know that men and women show accelerated signs of aging during flight. This is due in part to the lack of gravity. Because of this, space has become an effective model for aging, and we spend a great deal of time analyzing both what aging means for astronauts and how we can apply the information to medicine on Earth.

Another area we think about is the impact of sex and gender on human adaptation in space. Ultimately, if people live for an extended time in an orbiting space station or in a permanent structure on the moon, what will be their specific health concerns and how can we prepare for them? And what about sex?

SEX IN SPACE

When we talk about sending people to live in a permanent home in a space station or even on the moon, we have to talk about providing for basic human needs. When I think about the basic drives in all of us, I think of sleeping, eating and sex. There is a reason for these three, and it's survival of the species. We don't want to live without any of them. Deprivation of any of these drives leads either to death or to overindulgence once they're re-introduced.

Eating in space can be easily accommodated. Astronauts report a change in their ability to taste and prefer spicier or sweeter foods such as chocolate. Sleeping can be more problematic. Space travel contradicts one's natural inner clock. When you're experiencing sunrise and sunset every 90 minutes on board the International Space Station (ISS), the body doesn't regulate very easily. This aspect of space travel also affects production of hormones and neurotransmitters such as melatonin which can be involved in sleep.

Perhaps most interesting of all, however, is the idea of sex in space. Whenever I give a talk that uses "sex" and "space" in the title, it's a guarantee there will be more men in the room than usual. It's one way to get a captive audience. Imagine their reaction when they learn the talk is about the impact of sex and gender on health and adaptation during space travel.

On the other hand, if we're going to colonize the moon or visit a space "hotel," someone will eventually want to have sex. It's only our puritanical background that keeps us from discussing these issues. How will it work? One can assume the laws of physics will still apply—for every action there will be an equal and opposite reaction. That would be the first hurdle to overcome, especially in zero-g.

Many more questions remain to be answered. For example, how will contraception work? People in space lose some of their tactile sensations. How important is touch to the human body? We need gravity to develop and maintain strong bones and muscles. What will happen to offspring conceived in space? This question may now seem irrelevant to exploration, but if we are truly ever going to colonize distant worlds, it will be essential to survival.

These are all situations that need to be talked about on Earth as well. Can we ever afford to pretend sex won't always be an issue among humans? For example, look at the military and how many of our female sailors have become pregnant during the confines of a ship voyage. Some studies show that almost 10% of female sailors are lost to pregnancy. The U.S.S. Acadia during the first Gulf War in 1991 was dubbed the "Love Boat" by the press because 10% of its female crew, a total of 36 women, came home pregnant.

The numbers of pregnant women on the battlefield are not easy to obtain, but one report in 2003 revealed that the British in southern Iraq had to send 82 women home because they were pregnant. There's no denying that rules or no rules, programs or military guidelines, people will be driven to have sex, and we need to study its benefits and what happens if someone is denied this pleasure.

In the United States, we have politicized sex and in doing so have done a disservice to our health. Sexual health is a part of overall health. We have to be attuned to this and not view it as wrong in some way.

Look at the controversy over Plan B, a progestin-only emergency contraceptive pill. This pill is designed as an emergency contraceptive that can still prevent a pregnancy after contraceptive failure such as a condom breaking, unprotected sex, or rape. It doesn't stop a pregnancy that has already occurred, but prevents one from occurring as long as it is taken within 72 hours of unprotected sex.

About one woman in four feel nausea and about one in 17 vomits after taking Plan B. Otherwise, studies show it to be safe and effective and to reduce the risk of pregnancy by about 87-90 percent if taken within 72 hours of unprotected sex.

The controversy surrounding FDA approval of this medication being sold over the counter centers on the abortion issue. While some think that it equals abortion, I believe it's an effective tool giving women and girls control of their reproductive health, and that it actually prevents abortions. I also think we should give them credit that they will not use Plan B as a tool for contraception. There are side effects and I don't believe that women and girls will choose Plan B without thinking through all their options.

Consider that a woman or girl who is raped might take Plan B to prevent pregnancy. That same individual might have elected to have an abortion if a pregnancy did occur. Plan B does not act like an abortion drug, but rather like a preventive agent. Opponents of Plan B tried to keep it from being sold over-the-counter, effectively withholding the pill from women and girls who might have used it immediately following unprotected sex. Eventually the pill was approved for over-the-counter use for women over the age of 17, but not until it had been stigmatized with the word "abortion." In December 2011, Secretary Sebelius overruled the FDA decision to allow Plan B One-Step to be sold without a prescription to girls under the age of 17. Scientific data do not support this decision and it appears politically-based during an election year.

Another area where politics has interfered with science and health is sex education programs. In 2008, $204 million went to support programs that teach young people an abstinence-only curriculum concerning sex. This is opposed to programs that teach teens about safe-sex practices. There are studies that have shown that abstinence programs also gave young people a biased view of subjects such as the ineffectiveness of contraception or the risk of abortion in order to encourage them to avoid sex. They simply have not worked. I also think as a result, if some of these young people did choose to engage in sex, they wouldn't know how to talk with their partners about contraception or sexually transmitted diseases (STDs).

It is true that abstinence can technically prevent pregnancies and even STDs. However, we need to be truthful with our children about the evidence surrounding contraception. It reminds me of a letter to the editor I wrote in support of President Obama's campaign stance on reproductive health education. In it, I wrote of the struggles to use scientific evidence to ensure that reproductive health is considered a critical component of women's health. It frightens me to hear women say they are willing to sacrifice their right to choose what happens to their bodies in order to support a political ideal. It is concerning that policy and faith can erode the basic foundation supporting women's healthcare.

I came to this conclusion while working on a multi-million dollar embryo "adoption" program and an abstinence education program. Don't get me wrong. I believe faith has a place in healthcare. We need to appreciate that inner spirit; the love and the faith that surrounds a patient can impact their health and well-being. But faith should not dictate national policy.

After my letter was published, I received death threats. But I can't stay quiet on this issue. We should not mislead or distort reality to foster a climate of fear. We should encourage our children to ask questions and expect honest answers, to respect their bodies and to make decisions to protect their health and self-esteem.

There will always be peer pressure, but we do not have to add to the misconception surrounding sexual health. Parents as well as the healthcare community can play an important role to ensure that correct information is provided. I know it can be uncomfortable to engage children in conversations about sex, but we must do it.

BIKINI MEDICINE

I joined a meeting to discuss medical standards for the selection and retention of the astronaut corps, especially those going to the Moon, and possibly to Mars. The meeting had an air of urgency because traveling those distances, you can't hop in a taxi and come home if you become ill or disabled. Ideally, astronauts are healthy before they undertake the journey, but what constitutes healthy?

There's no question we've made great strides since the era of *The Right Stuff*, Tom Wolfe's account of the early days of space travel when astronauts could only be male fighter pilots. Astronauts at the beginning of the space program had no way of knowing what the effects of space travel might be on the human body.

I once sat at dinner with Senator John Glenn after he returned from his last space mission. Naturally our conversation got around to health in space. He told me that when he joined NASA, leading up to his Mercury 6 space flight in 1962, doctors weren't entirely sure if changes in pressure might make an astronaut's eyeballs pop out. Forty-some years later, we're still studying finely-tuned effects on the human body from long duration space travel.

What is the best age for people to undertake space exploration? We know there's an increased risk of cancer among astronauts because there is no atmosphere to offer protection from solar and cosmic radiation. I often mused whether we should let older people rather than younger people assume that risk since the latency period for the development of cancer can be quite long. Ill effects might not be seen in older astronauts because they could die before the cancers show up.

There have been discussions surrounding the reproductive health of astronauts. During one conversation, the question arose should a woman be excluded from space travel if she has endometriosis? This is a condition where tissue similar to the lining of the uterus shows up elsewhere in a woman's body, mainly in the abdominal cavity, and can be the cause of pelvic discomfort, especially around the time of one's period. Over five million women in the United States have this condition, which so far is incurable, but can certainly be treated.

During this discussion, it appeared there was consensus that if a woman could be treated for endometriosis, she could stay in the space program. This discussion reminded me of a comment that I once heard from a colleague.

"Well," he said. "After all, a woman doesn't need a uterus to fly the space shuttle."

I know that this was meant to be a joke and to lighten the tension in a conversation which it did achieve.

"Okay," I said to myself in the same jocular vein, "Do men need prostate glands or testes to fly? Why don't we just cut them out as well as long as we're going to view women in terms of body parts and not the whole person?"

For me, this type of dialogue triggered a familiar frustration with attitudes toward women's health. While there is still a long way to go, I want to be optimistic that we can get there.

Historically, a woman's anatomy was thought to be an inferior version of a man's. Overall, nothing received as much suspicion as the uterus, which medical practitioners in the middle ages believed to be a distinctly female organ that caused a host of specifically female diseases. The term "hysteria" comes from the Greek word for uterus. Hysteria was described as a condition in which a woman's womb wandered at will throughout the body. At its most vicious, the uterus was thought to migrate upwards and cut off the very breath of life. No male organ could be found that affected the body so dramatically.

Women prone to hysteria (with its enormous list of symptoms such as nervousness, irritability and a tendency to cause trouble) were treated in various ways. One approach, which seems almost unbelievable today, was a late 19th century practice in which a physician provided manual stimulation or massage of the clitoris with a vibrator until the woman was "cured by an orgasm." Eventually in the early 1900s, the pornography industry took an interest in vibrators, and they moved from medicinal purposes into the realm of sexual practices.

In the mid 20th century, the medical profession moved past the idea of hysteria and came to view women as a collection of body parts especially breasts, vagina, uterus and ovaries. This was called "bikini medicine." In the beginning, it raised the level of awareness that men and women were different. But it took it to a point where it became disparaging to women because it covered only the body parts that were covered by a bikini. That mindset still stays with us and it's hard to penetrate through that. It was the easy way out. When we're looking at the brain, lungs and heart, we have to dig deeper.

As medical care continued to evolve, the profession built specialty clinics in women's health such as bone health, heart health and reproductive health. Unfortunately, there was often no communication between clinics and healthcare became more fragmented. At the same time, women's health service lines developed to act as marketing tools to increase clinic and hospital revenues. While most of these services are reproductive based, they also include cosmetic or spa treatments as an incentive to encourage women to schedule appointments.

I believe that it's now time to take a step forward and approach women's health in a multi-disciplinary, comprehensive way, viewing each woman as a whole person, and not just separate parts. At the beginning of the 21st century, we're finally developing the field of sex and gender-based medicine that pays attention to specific differences and similarities between men and women. This exciting area of science was pioneered by Dr. Florence Haseltine and Phyllis Greenberger, founders of The Society for Women's Health Research and Dr. Vivian Pinn, the first director of The Office of Research on Women's Health at the National Institutes of Health. In order to provide the most effective healthcare, we have to continue emphasizing both an integrative approach to medicine as well as gender and sex-specific studies.

Sometimes the public and even the doctors underestimate the need for a uterus which reflects an old way of thinking. Today, can we really be cavalier about whether a woman needs her uterus, when reproductive health is integral to overall health, and vice versa? The health of the uterus is a key issue women face, and we can hardly relegate it to the status of a vestigial organ. I support that we view reproductive health as an essential component to women's health. You cannot advance women's health without protecting reproductive health.

According to an article in the *New England Journal of Medicine*, hysterectomies are the second most common major operation in the United States; ironically the first is cesarean sections. By the age of 60, over a third of women in the United States have had a hysterectomy. According to one study, over 50 percent of hospital stays related to endometriosis resulted in abdominal hysterectomy.

Let me give an example of how I would approach a woman with endometriosis if she were my patient. As a doctor specializing in women's health, I want my patient to protect and keep her uterus as long as possible. The decision to remove it should be seen in the light of her overall well-being. Certainly it would be a start if she understood the role of the uterus in her body, some of the most common problems affecting the organ, and some of the alternatives for treatment.

Even after childbearing years, the uterus does not become as expendable as an appendix, for instance. I've been astounded to learn that after a hysterectomy, many women don't even know what exactly was removed from their bodies, or if part of their uterus, ovaries or cervix were left after the surgery.

During my work in medical schools, I've discovered that a lot of interns may use the term hysterectomy, but not know what parts of the uterus were removed and what was left behind. We've become nonchalant about hysterectomies, but it's a significant surgical procedure with risks and complications. This is basic healthcare, and yet so many people don't know how to put it in context.

A lot of doctors look at the uterus as the cause of endometriosis which again is due to uterine or endometrial tissue outside the uterus. A hysterectomy does not treat the uterine tissue outside the uterus that may be causing the pain. In some cases, a procedure using a tube with a camera on the end which is called laparoscopy may find only a small amount of the disease, but the patient may nonetheless be experiencing severe pain. Another woman may have a lot of tissue outside the uterus, but not be symptomatic at all. Many women are unsure of what's causing pain, and the only way to truly diagnose the condition is during surgery.

Clearly, there is not just one treatment for this disease. A too simplistic view can do a disservice to our patients. The beauty of women's health is its complexity. To unravel it and treat our patients is our task.

Endometriosis can actually get better on its own with age, or it can be treated medically with hormonal manipulation. For example, drugs that chemically induce menopause or contraceptives, decreasing cyclic menstrual changes which impact endometrial tissue inside or outside the uterus, may decrease pain. Another treatment is to shut down the hormonal supply to this tissue by removing the ovaries, thus surgically inducing menopause. If it becomes apparent that a woman should absolutely have her uterus and/or ovaries removed, the next step is to define exactly what is going to be removed and what is left behind. All of this should be undertaken with caution and a view to overall health.

Before having any organ removed from the body, I would advise a woman facing a hysterectomy to first ask herself how much confidence she has in her doctor and then know the risks and benefits, understand alternative procedures, and always remember that she can ask for another opinion. We are all our own best advocates in a doctor's office, and we should feel comfortable about bringing a friend or family member who can take notes and be a sounding board.

In the long run, I am glad to be part of NASA's discussions concerning health in space. Again, the extreme laboratory of space travel highlights the most basic questions about men's and women's health. At the end of the day, what parts of our bodies do we need to live a good life and to do our jobs? Can we really take out organs without affecting the health of our whole being? Would a man agree to have his prostate gland or a testicle removed for his career? Viewed from that perspective, doesn't it seem absurd to view women as a collection of expendable body parts?

At the same time, I don't believe it's up to our government to dictate sexual behavior from a moralistic standpoint, but rather for the government to fund research studies and examine the results leading to effective policies. Controversial reproductive health issues should be viewed from the standpoint of scientific evidence and basic health, not from the viewpoint of right or wrong. Our lives on Earth and in space depend on this balanced approach.

Sometimes even our own health can get lost in this world of split-second media and political medicine. Maybe a fresh perspective, such as one from the moon looking down at the blue oceans of the Earth, can help us see the truth more clearly. In the future, there could be sex in space. But for now, I doubt there is much use for a bikini.

Stellar Questions:

Is there a demographic aspect to hysterectomies?

Studies show that more women in the south received hysterectomies and at an earlier age than in the north (eight out of 1000 women in the south vs. five out of 1000 in the north). This data may point to racial inequities that exist in healthcare in the United States. It may be that some doctors aren't looking at alternative therapies or that women aren't asking for them. Sometimes the most radical treatment doesn't need to be done. Never do something unless you feel completely comfortable. Some questions to ask yourself about your medical care include: How do they treat me? Are my calls being returned on time? Is information being explained in a way that I can understand?

Can I freeze my ovaries for later use?

This process remains in an experimental phase. It requires small tissue from the ovaries, and has yielded only a few hundred live births so far. Although sperm and embryo freezing has been commonplace, egg cells often don't survive the freezing and thawing process because the water in these cells forms ice crystals which can destroy the eggs during the process.

I have frozen my embryos, but I don't want more children, what can I do with these embryos?

There are basically four options: maintain them, destroy them, donate them to scientific research for stem cell studies, or provide them for embryo donation. Over a million dollars of taxpayer money has gone into programs to facilitate embryo donation. Some of these federally funded programs have used the term "adoption" instead of "donation." It's important to know that there are approximately 400,000 embryos in storage in the U.S., but many may not be healthy enough to become babies. Of those under five years in storage, about one in ten might grow into a full term baby. Don't let the term "adoption" force you to think that every embryo represents a future baby. I believe this is the abortion debate under another disguise. What you do with frozen embryos is your decision, which should be made carefully.

Should I let my daughter get vaccinated with the cervical cancer vaccine?

The human papilloma vaccine is designed to immunize young women against cervical cancer, genital warts, and sexually transmitted diseases (STDs) caused by the Human Papilloma Virus (HPV). There are 37 types of the virus that are transmitted through sexual contact. Most come and go without symptoms, but 19 represent high-risk types that can lead to cancers. The Merck HPV vaccine targets the two most high-risk viruses that cause 70 percent of cervical cancer. The first HPV vaccine was approved in June 2006 for 9 to 26-year-old girls and women. The vaccine won't prevent every cancer and infection of the cervix. It is not effective if there has already been exposure to HPV. Pelvic exams and PAP smears are still important as well as safe sexual practices. Some have thought that this vaccine gives girls permission to have sex. I believe it helps girls be safe from a potentially life-threatening disease.

Are there dietary aspects to PMS?

Premenstrual syndrome (PMS) affects women of childbearing age. The cause is unknown, but it is most likely due to fluctuating levels of hormones. The symptoms can include bloating, breast tenderness, unexpected weeping, headaches, food cravings, fatigue, anxiety and depression. Evidence shows that up to 85% of pre-menopausal women experience these symptoms. PMS can be treated with medications, exercise and nutrition. Studies show that by reducing your intake of caffeine, salt and sugar and increasing your intake of foods that would yield 1200 mg of calcium per day (yogurt, milk or cheese) can improve the condition. In some cases, nutritional supplements such as vitamins B6, D, E, and magnesium have also been effective. As always, drinking 8-10 glasses of water every day, limiting your alcohol consumption and adding Omega 3 fatty acids found in fatty fish such as salmon may improve your ability to handle this syndrome.

Is it okay to suppress my periods for many months?

An adjustment of your menstrual cycle allows you to have less frequent periods and to avoid bleeding at inconvenient times. In the big picture it may also help manage conditions like endometriosis. Suppression may reduce painful, heavy periods and menstrual migraines. Among the major disadvantages of suppression is an increase of breakthrough bleeding in the first few cycles. The risks accompanying this include blood clots, heart attacks and strokes, which are seen with all oral contraceptives. There are those who say the menstrual cycle should be considered a vital sign just like blood pressure checks. If women are stressed or underweight, they might not have a period. How long can a woman safely continue on a pill that suppresses their menses? There is approved medication for suppression up to 12 weeks.

Can a woman over 50 get AIDS?

The Centers for Disease Control and Prevention (CDC) reports that AIDS cases in Americans over fifty rose from 16,300 in 1995, to 90,600 in 2003. They also report that women over fifty represent 18% of the AIDS cases, which is one of the fastest growing groups. One aspect of this is that menopause can lead to thinning and dryness in the vaginal wall which causes small rips with sex that might increase AIDS transmission. More than half of those infected over fifty are African-American and Hispanic. Older women have higher incidence than older men. I believe health providers fall into the trap of AIDS stereotypes, and don't provide the prevention information to older Americans that would help them prevent this disease.

My mother, who is widowed, is now dating, so how do I talk to her about sex?

This is a continuation of the issue of women and AIDS. Older people in America tend to view condoms as simply a way to prevent pregnancy. Studies show that only one in six people over fifty might use condoms. In general, older people have less basic knowledge about HIV prevention and STDs. I believe we need an overall reduction in the stigma of sexual needs in older people and an increase in sexual discussion. In essence, we have blinders on. It's important to discuss with your mother or any other older person the consequences of AIDS and STDs. I know this isn't easy, but you might try using a pamphlet as an ice-breaker. These pamphlets often lie in retirement centers or doctors' offices. There are many organizations and community centers devoted to providing information for older women. The bottom line is you can't be shy to encourage an older person to talk with her partner about these issues. Tell them to ask for a sexual history. Sometimes, being with a man who has an erection might be so exciting, you don't ask about a sexual history, but men can carry infections and not even know it. Don't forget that a bit of humor can often help break the ice in this type of conversation.

Is there Viagra for women?

Viagra is a drug for men that increases blood flow to the penis so that there is an erection. Although a drug like Viagra could increase blood flow to the clitoris and the vagina in a woman, it doesn't necessarily mean an increase in desire. There is a difference between genital changes and mental stimulation. With women, there are many more factors involved in sexual satisfaction. Many companies have looked for the magic bullet for women and are testing patches of hormones such as testosterone, but nothing has been approved yet. I think that the best aphrodisiac for a woman is the seduction that first stimulates her heart and mind rather than her genitals.

Can a woman get pregnant after she goes through menopause?

I have thought of this question as should we have nurseries next to our nursing homes? Yes, a woman can get pregnant during the "process" of menopause. Perimenopause is a time of irregular periods that can last five to ten years, and you can get pregnant during this time because ovulation can still occur.

When you've not had a period for more than a year, then you have gone through menopause. We generally think a woman is safe from pregnancy after menopause, but it's still important to practice safe sex to prevent STDs. There is also an opportunity for women to get pregnant after menopause if they have a healthy uterus, for instance by receiving a donated egg that has been fertilized by in vitro fertilization. There are women over sixty who have had pregnancies this way.

Generally, they are in good health and closely followed. Nevertheless, there are lots of ethical questions such as will the child have a mother who is too old to raise a child? Interestingly, these questions are often not asked about men at the same age. Older sperm can carry genetic defects in the same way that older eggs can. With our current technology, nurseries next to nursing homes may be a reality, but are they smart?

CHAPTER FOUR
GLOBAL WARMING AND MORE HOT FLASHES
—A Time for Menopause

"I have enjoyed greatly the second blooming…
suddenly you find—at the age of 50, say—
that a whole new life has opened before you."

—Agatha Christie

I once held a town hall meeting on menopause on Capitol Hill. I invited interesting and well-respected speakers to educate lawmakers and their staff, federal employees, diplomats and their spouses and healthcare professionals on the latest information surrounding this monumental time in a woman's life known as menopause. Two moments stand out the most. I recall Dr. Marilyn Gaston, the former Assistant Surgeon General talk about hot flashes. She said that if we thought that there was global warming now, we should just wait until all the baby boomers reach the age of menopause. That got a big laugh.

During lunch, we had the first appearance of a performance from Menopause the Musical in Washington, D.C. I will never forget the embarrassed looks on the congressmen's faces as the performers sang about sex and hot flashes all in one breath. It is interesting to see what makes Congress blush. Perhaps some were having their own hot flashes.

There is one thing I want to get across about menopause—it is not a disease. It is as naturally a part of life as puberty. It is also not new. Had women in previous centuries not died during childbirth or pandemics, they would have experienced menopause as we do now.

In today's world, menopause has been capitalized and not just because I took it to Capitol Hill. It is used to sell hormonal therapies, blood tests, and even clothing and head wear. It is no longer seen as a phase of life but as a branded part of a marketing plan. The medical industry is no different. There are medical organizations that actually offer certification to become Menopause Clinicians and Menopause Educators. Physicians can be deemed specialists in menopause. Imagine if we called pediatricians "puberty specialists" if they also took an additional course. The bottom line is that menopause sells!

* * *

One study represents the cornerstone to menopause research. The National Institutes of Health launched the Women's Health Initiative in 1991 to study health issues affecting post-menopausal women. It was the largest study ever undertaken. The most dramatic findings occurred in 2002 when the estrogen plus progesterone trial ended abruptly when investigators found the subjects showed an increased risk for coronary heart disease, breast cancer and strokes.

At the time, I received advance notice the night before that the National Institutes of Health was making a major announcement in the morning. I got to the National Press Club early and sat down in the front row next to a number of my colleagues. When the findings were shared, I had one thought. I was glad I was not in private practice any more. I knew my phones would have been ringing off the hook.

In the end, the message of the Women's Health Initiative was that hormones were potentially dangerous. To be fair, there was some good in the report, but all that was forgotten. Once the findings were announced, an uproar raged across the nation. Women everywhere were afraid. They wondered what they had been doing to themselves all those years taking hormone replacement therapy or as we now call it "Menopausal Hormone Therapy" or "MHT" since hormones did not technically need to be replaced to be healthy.

Over the next few months, I worked with the FDA and others to craft a message to the public. The FDA wanted to provide factual information to help guide women toward making educated decisions. It was not as easy as "hormones are bad." They also had to generate a statement that applied to all sex hormones even though only one regimen was used. This generalization already made the statement slightly inaccurate, but we had to keep it simple. We recommended that if women needed to take hormones for hot flashes or vaginal dryness that they use the smallest dosage for the shortest amount of time. Most assumed that it would ideally be for less than two years.

When I was in private practice, I remember having patients who were debilitated by lack of sleep caused by night sweats. They swore that hormone therapy gave them their lives back. No matter what reaction it caused, the study did open the debate—a debate that needed to be aired to the public. Prior to the initiative, hormone replacement therapy was considered to be the great elixir of life. In the 1960s, a book was published, *Feminine Forever* by Dr. Robert Wilson, that extolled the virtues of the therapy. It was a best seller and probably did a lot to increase the popularity of the treatment. Now, the possible dangers of the treatment were on the front page of newspapers across the country. Because of that, women started to personalize their own medical care. It also showed women that even if they started something like hormone therapy; it did not mean they had to continue it forever.

The downside, however, was that women thought they had been hurting themselves for years. Some women's health advocates came forward and said that there was never a need to use hormone therapy; and that it represented the corruption of the medical and scientific community by industry. Doctors are still dealing with the backlash from the mistrust the results fostered.

The bottom line is that there is not one simple answer. What works well for your friend or your sister might not work for you. As you age, what worked for you one day might not the next. We are dynamic beings and the medical system has to adjust to that. So my best advice is to ask questions and educate yourself.

* * *

I will never forget the first talk that I gave on menopause. I was a fellow in endocrinology at the University of California, San Francisco (UCSF) and the speech was to my college alumni group. The other speakers were UCSF professors who were there to talk about cardiovascular health and depression during menopause. I was just a first year fellow at that time, so I was a little intimidated being at the table with them.

The funny thing was that we were in a garage, literally. It was one of the alumni member's houses. I was there standing next to a tool chest and a car talking about estrogen and progesterone. Even at the time, I found the venue funny. Not in its informality but in its utter maleness.

It was in that garage that I found my calling. I loved every minute of it. I got an enormous rush, the same rush I'd get later in life talking to much larger crowds. I felt like I shared information and my audience really understood it.

That talk spurred me on to want to take care of women going through menopause. It changed the direction of my career; a true epiphany moment in a garage in San Francisco. I completed my first year in endocrinology. Then, I also did a fellowship in geriatrics at the same time as my endocrinology fellowship because back then women going through menopause were considered "old." During that time, I designed and completed a women's health fellowship by going beyond endocrinology and geriatrics. I went to many departments to inquire if I could work with them to see patients and help with clinical trials.

By the end of the fellowship which was the first in the nation in women's health, I was supported by general and reproductive endocrinology, obstetrics and gynecology, geriatrics, cardiology and radiology. I think that I had three days off the first year, but I learned so much and loved every minute of it. All of it led to my dream of helping women through what to some is considered a disease, others a business opportunity, but to me a natural course of life—menopause.

By definition, menopause starts 12 months from the time of your last period. Changes, however, start before that time. It is not a light switch. Your period will, or has, probably slowed in regularity before it stops. Symptoms can come on years before your final menstruation. Changing hormone levels may be the cause for the early symptoms of menopause called perimenopause. The level of estrogen, progesterone and androgens (male hormones) all change as your body waltzes out of your reproductive years. By the time a year has passed since your last period, menopause is considered over. Like everything else in life, it is not quite that simple.

SYMPTOMS

No two women have the exact same experience with perimenopause or menopause. As estrogen levels decrease, changes can occur throughout the body. Here are a few common symptoms and why they occur:

Menstrual Changes: The most obvious but less often spoken signs are menstrual changes. This is the keystone to menopause. As previously mentioned, the definition of menopause is based on a women's final period. During perimenopause, your period may become irregular. It can be more intense, or less; longer or shorter. Some changes should be watched more closely. If your periods come too close together or last more than a week, you should check with your doctor. That may not be a symptom of menopause but an issue with the lining of your uterus.

Hot Flashes: This is the most infamous symptom of menopause. It seems to be the butt of every joke involving aging women. Hot flashes are a sudden rush of heat, usually felt in the upper body. It can be accompanied by rapid heartbeat, sweating, dizziness, nausea, headache and a general malaise. It is followed often by a flushing of the face and neck.

Most likely, they are caused by a change in estrogen levels. A lower level of estrogen can affect the hypothalamus. It is the area of your brain that helps control body temperature. Whatever the level of estrogen does to the brain, it seems to cause wires to get crossed, making the body think it is too hot. It reacts by dilating blood vessels and triggering sweat glands to dissipate the falsely identified heat.

Most women experience some level of hot flashes during perimenopause and menopause. The intensity and duration of the flashes can vary greatly. Strangely, it has been found that the most common times hot flashes are suffered are between six and eight in the morning and six and ten at night. Ironically, this is around the time that men's testosterone levels increase which stimulate their libido. Nature has a strange sense of humor—both sexes are hot, but in very different ways!

Mood Swings: Mood swings are another common symptom of menopause. Once again, they are caused by hormonal changes. Similar symptoms are common among pregnant women. Fatigue from insomnia, perhaps from night sweats, can cause mood swings and irritability.

Obviously, your mood can be affected by psychological factors as well. For many people, changes in their lives can cause emotional responses that lead to irritability. Your mind might be abuzz with thoughts and concerns, making it hard to focus on the everyday bumps in life. Now, when that change is your own body, it is no wonder your mood might swing. Think of a teenager going through puberty. Maybe it is not so different.

Insomnia: Sleep can be an elusive treasure during perimenopause. It is no wonder irritability is a symptom as well. Nothing can affect the mood more strongly than sleep deprivation.

The cause of insomnia during menopause is uncertain. Some researchers have tied it to low levels of estrogen. Others have pointed to other causes, some psychological, some nutritional.

Sex: Many women find that their sex life changes with menopause. The change, however, is not the same for everyone. Some women find themselves less interested; some more. For some, the knowledge that they cannot become pregnant adds a new dimension of freedom to their life. Also, by the age of menopause, most women have grown children that are out of the house, or at least less dependent, allowing them to relax and enjoy their sex life. For others, issues such as vaginal dryness hamper their enjoyment of sex. Although water-soluble lubricants are a simple solution, the discomfort or embarrassment of vaginal dryness can still lessen intimacy.

Once again, estrogen is one possible cause, but not the only one. Other changes to a women's body as she ages can affect sex drive such as bladder control, medication and other health issues, and sleep disturbances. One thing seems certain to me. All the signs and symptoms of menopause are tied together. They are all a part of the change our bodies are going through and should be considered as a unit.

TREATMENT

Looking at all the signs and symptoms together, many may be traced back to changes in hormone levels. It is no wonder that hormone therapy is a common treatment for menopause. It is not the only option though. Other treatments are available:

Hormone Therapy: It is believed that many of the symptoms common in menopause occur when estrogen levels decrease. Estrogen is still one of the most effective treatments of menopausal symptoms such as hot flashes and night sweats. Although it is no longer routinely recommended for long-term use, short-term use has been shown to be potentially beneficial. Some studies have found that it may help reduce the risk of heart disease if taken early during menopause. Yet, other studies show that MHT may increase the risk of heart events in some women. This is where personalized medicine using genetic profiling in the future may be able to show which women could have deleterious or beneficial effects.

Hormone therapy is definitely not for everyone. In 2002, the Women's Health Initiative found that hormone therapy can be more dangerous than beneficial. They looked at a group of 10,000 women who took a combination of estrogen and progestin, a synthetic progesterone, compared to a control group that were given a placebo. They found an increased risk of heart disease, including mortality rates, breast cancer, stroke and blood clots in the group who took MHT. The increased risk was small when looking at a single woman's risk, but as a group, it was enough to consider it a public health concern.

The study also evaluated women who only used estrogen therapy. There were 23 percent fewer breast cancer cases and 46 percent fewer heart attacks if they started therapy close to menopause. Unfortunately, the risk of strokes and blood clots did not change. In the end, the study showed that hormone therapy was not the silver bullet it was once considered to be.

There is another option for hormone treatment that has gained a great deal of attention. It is called bio-identical hormone therapy. In essence, these are hormones that identically match those made by the human body. Some are made just as other drugs are, but some are produced by special "compounding" pharmacies. At these pharmacies, the prescription is made specifically for each patient. But keep in mind that the receptors on cells in the body only see the drug as a hormone and it does not register that it is synthetic or bio—identical and thus the risks may be similar.

Symptom-specific Treatments: Many doctors may choose to treat the specific symptom that is most troubling to their patient. For hot flashes, an anti-seizure medication, Gabapentin, has been found to lessen their frequency. In addition, Clonidine, a blood pressure medicine, has shown some signs of helping to lessen the discomfort associated with hot flashes, but it has also been known to cause undesirable side effects, specifically hypotension (low blood pressure) that can be fatal. Anti-depressants have been used in low dosages to help with hot flashes as well. Each woman responds differently and at different dosages.

Vaginal estrogen and selective estrogen receptor modulators (SERMS) have shown some promise to be more selective in their responses while minimizing side effects. Vaginal estrogen is a local dose of the hormone, usually administered through cream or an insertable tablet that can help prevent vaginal dryness which can lead to irritation, painful intercourse and a higher risk of urinary tract infections. SERMs have been shown to prevent bone density loss. They may pose less risk than regular estrogen because they act differently in different tissue. SERMS do not decrease hot flashes and for some women, there may even be an increase.

ALTERNATIVE THERAPY

At the beginning of this century, hormone therapy was a common prescription to women during menopause. Not only did it reduce some annoying symptoms, but it also helped prevent osteoporosis. Interestingly, even before the Women's Health Initiative's findings on the risks of hormone therapy, only 35-40 percent of women ever started taking hormones for menopause. Many of those discontinued the therapy early. Why was this the case?

Perhaps they felt that hormone therapy did not feel natural. Now, with the known risks, even more women are looking for other methods to help alleviate symptoms related to menopause, and many are turning to alternative therapies.

Physical Activity: Some researches think that unregulated levels of the neurotransmitter, norepinephrine, could initiate hot flashes. Moderate exercise has been shown to increase central opioid activity in the brain and increase the sense of well-being—a natural high which may help alleviate hot flashes. In one study done in 1990, researchers found that activity levels decreased the severity of the episodes, but not the frequency. Unfortunately, this study had some limitations when it came to isolating physical activity as the sole influence. Another study showed that only five percent of women who exercised regularly experienced severe hot flashes compared to 15 percent of those who were not as active.

Although there is still too little data to make the absolute statement that physical activity alleviates hot flashes, it is hard to ignore the overall health benefit exercise provides you. Whether you do it to control the severity of menopausal symptoms or for weight control or heart health, the overall benefits far outweigh the potential risks. As always, check with your doctor before beginning a new exercise regime.

Vitamin E: Some studies have alluded that vitamin E may reduce hot flashes as well. One study used a placebo-controlled trial and found a marginal benefit from ingesting 800 IU of vitamin E daily.

So far, research has not conclusively proven that vitamin E can help control menopausal symptoms. At the same time, ingesting too much of the vitamin has been proven to be a bad idea. It can lead to muscle fatigue, nausea and diarrhea. It can also react poorly if you are taking an anticoagulant such as Warfarin.

Soy: Soy is a popular alternative medicine for the symptoms of menopause. It contains phytoestrogen, which is a plant derivative with mild estrogenic and anti-estrogenic properties. Flaxseed is another food that is high in phytoestrogen.

An interesting cultural variance excited researchers in this area. Women in Asia rarely report menopausal symptoms. Why? One reason may be that they eat more soy. Unfortunately, research has not isolated soy as the only reason. There are other cultural differences, such as Asian women being less likely to admit such symptoms that could account for the difference or they may describe it as shoulder pain rather than a hot flash.

Another study looked at the claims that high soy diets can provide similar results as estrogen therapy. Although they found that the medical evidence supports the health benefits of phytoestrogens, the science shows that conventional estrogen therapy is far more effective.

At the same time, a study done in 1998 found a significant reduction in hot flashes among women treated with soy, 45 percent compared to 30 percent for the control group. As long as you are careful, a diet with moderate amounts of soy can't hurt your health. Although there are over-the-counter supplements available, the best way to increase your intake is through food. Soy milk and tofu are great options. There is no general agreement to how much soy you need to ingest to get any benefits. Additionally, studies are underway to see if phytoestrogens are related to the same health concerns as other estrogens produced in the body or the synthetic variety.

Bodywork: Bodywork therapies include acupuncture, massage and chiropractic manipulation. In 1996, a large health maintenance organization (HMO) found that these therapies were the most common alternative treatments used by their members.

More and more, women are turning to alternative medicine to treat their menopausal symptoms. In 2002, a study from Washington State surveyed women between the age of 45 and 65, asking them if they used a number of alternative therapies. They found that 22 percent of the women surveyed used at least one of eight different alternative treatments and that of them, nearly 100 percent found them to be "somewhat or very helpful."

Much like exercise, bodywork therapy may help hot flashes by increasing opioid activity. One recent study, however, found little actual benefit. They conducted a single-blind (meaning the researcher already knew the particular group), sham-controlled clinical trial on women already suffering hot flashes. After six weeks, there was little difference between the subjects receiving actual medical acupuncture and those receiving a sham version, an acupuncture version of a placebo. The jury on alternative treatments is still out on the effectiveness of alternative or what may be called traditional therapies.

THE BUSINESS OF MENOPAUSE

According to a *New York Times* article by Karen Stabiner in 1998, the alternate health remedy industry was a $4 billion business. After the WHI study, many women turned in this direction to treat menopausal symptoms. With this, products claiming to "cure" menopause flooded the market.

When you talk about the business of menopause, it is hard to ignore Suzanne Somers. She has been in the limelight discussing this issue for some time. She came out as a vocal proponent of bio-identical hormones, specifically in her book, *Ageless: The Naked Truth about Bioidentical Hormones*. This treatment claims to provide hormonal replacement that matches the natural hormone production in the ovaries. In some ways, she brings back the themes of Dr. Robert Wilson's *Feminine Forever*, implying that bio-identical hormones might help women stay younger longer.

Along with bio-identical hormones and herbal supplements, other products are available. Many women suffer night sweats during menopause. In many cases, these occurrences are significant enough to soak through the sufferer's clothing. The damp clothes than can lead to interrupted sleep. Some companies have developed night clothes that are made of the same kinds of material as running apparel. The fabric is specially designed to pull moisture away from the skin.

Another product is an at-home hormone test kit. Much like pregnancy tests, these products claim to let a women know when she is going through menopause. Some of the tests are FDA approved. There are urine and saliva tests that look at the levels of certain hormones produced by the pituitary gland such as follicle-stimulating hormone or FSH, that tend to increase as a women nears menopause.

Just as in pregnancy tests, it is probably a better idea to go to your doctor. At the same time, menopause, although natural, is different than pregnancy. In my opinion, if you don't have menopausal symptoms, than buying a home test to find out may not be the best use of your money. Perhaps it is better to spend your time and money living a healthy lifestyle with good nutrition, exercise, stress reduction and sleep.

* * *

It's funny. There is so much misunderstanding when it comes to menopause. It reminds me of my first experience with it. When I was around ten, my mother had a hysterectomy. She had uterine fibroids. Due to a family history of ovarian cancer, her doctor decided to remove her ovaries as a precaution.

After surgery, I was sitting in the hospital room with my mom when her doctor came in to talk to her. I remember him saying that because he took her ovaries, she should be careful of what she ate because she would likely put on weight. With that, he walked out of the room.

Within days of surgery, my mom who was in her early 40s started to experience symptoms of menopause. She started complaining about being hot. She got tired quickly and she wasn't sleeping well. She said she was hungry all the time and did put on weight. It was such an immediate change; it amazed me.

Being a child, I latched onto what I heard that doctor say. My young mind came to the obvious conclusion. Menopause was going to make me fat. That, coupled with the other symptoms I saw my mom suffer, I thought menopause was a horrific thing, a black hole you fall into when you loose your ovaries.

Although in an exaggerated way, the story of my childhood understanding of the disease is so much like the struggle women go through as they approach menopause. There is fear and confusion about what to do. At the same time, most of the fear can be alleviated simply by education. Find a good doctor and ask a lot of questions. Get yourself ready so that when the time comes, you'll have the tools to make good decisions that will help you. Remember, there is no silver bullet. That's okay, though, because menopause is not a disease. It is part of life.

When you go into perimenopause, you should evaluate your health. If, to preserve your quality of life, you need treatment, you should talk to your doctor about possible risk factors for diseases such as heart disease, stroke, cancer, dementia and osteoporosis and your risks associated with menopausal treatments. You should know your family history and risk factors. Only then can you decide what you may want to do.

What will I do when I get menopause? I always say I will go to the space station and see if microgravity helps hot flashes. In reality, I can't tell you yet. I won't know until I experience it and come up with an individual plan that will best suit me and what I am experiencing. You can be sure though that I will ask questions and be open to many different approaches since there is not one perfect path. But most importantly, living a healthy lifestyle will top the list. Much like the cars in that garage where I gave my first talk on menopause, our bodies need to be maintained, occasionally tuned up and always revered.

Stellar Questions

What is the difference between natural menopause and surgical menopause?

Sometimes menopause is not a natural progression of a woman's life. When a hysterectomy is required, the doctor may also remove both ovaries. This is called a bilateral oophorectomy. This procedure may be necessary in cases of ovarian cysts or cancer.

When both ovaries are removed, menopause will ensue. This varies from the non-surgical menopause, which is a natural sequence of events. In the case of surgical menopause, because the change occurs instantaneously, the symptoms can be more pronounced or appear more severe. Compounding the problem, women with surgical menopause may be younger, adding another psychological factor to the equation. Also, they are in the process of recovering from major surgery, and may be dealing with a life threatening illness if the ovaries were removed due to disease.

What can cause premature menopause?

As mentioned above, surgical menopause is considered premature menopause when it occurs before the age of 40, but other factors can cause a woman's body to change before the typical age range. Sometimes, even if the ovaries are left intact after a hysterectomy, blood flow can be interrupted, thus creating the same effect as surgical menopause. As long as you have one ovary that is functioning normally, you can still have your menstrual cycle. Without a uterus, you may not have withdrawal bleeding so knowing you are going through menopause could be more difficult.

Another condition is sometimes considered as premature menopause or premature ovarian failure that may be related to antibodies against the ovaries—it is like an autoimmune disease and can be a cause of infertility as well.

In addition to premature ovarian failure, other factors could cause "premature menopause." Chemotherapy and thyroid disorders can cause premature menopause. Regardless, if you are under 40 and begin showing signs of premature menopause—irregular periods, hot flashes, vaginal dryness, etc—see your doctor.

What is the difference between natural and synthetic hormones?

There are "natural" alternatives to MHT. Estrogen and progesterone can be made from food such as soy and yams. Sometimes these are called bio—identical hormones. People are drawn to this natural option because they can be made to mirror the hormones a woman's body would produce naturally prior to menopause.

One big difference between natural and synthetic is that the FDA does not regulate natural hormones. A potential advantage of bio-identical hormones is that they are individualized as opposed to one-size-fits-all drug. It is important to note that receptors and cells in the body will probably not recognize whether the hormones being introduced are natural or synthetic. It is widely accepted that high levels of any form of estrogen can increase risk for uterine and breast cancer.

What plants are sources of natural hormones?

Soy is often considered a possible "natural" treatment for menopausal symptoms. It contains phytoestrogens. As the name implies, these are estrogen like substances extracted from a plant. Keep in mind, the science is spotty when it comes to the efficacy of soy as a treatment for symptoms such as hot flashes.

Yams and black cohosh are also mentioned as possible treatments for menopausal symptoms, but definitive conclusions are difficult to reach concerning their usefulness as a treatment. The available data showed no consistent reduction in the severity of hot flashes with black cohosh. Wild yams are another source often discussed. They are hypothesized to contain properties than can act like the precursor to estrogen and progesterone. It is believed that one would need to eat an entire truckload of yams to get to therapeutic levels. Products derived from plants are not known to be 100 percent safe which surprises many. Nor is it proven that they are an effective treatment for menopause. Before using any plant-based supplement, make sure you speak to your doctor.

Can hormone therapy be given orally on the skin?

Both estrogen and progesterone can be delivered to the body in different methods. Estrogen can come in a pill, a skin patch, vaginal ring insert or shot. Similarly, progesterone can come in a pill, patch, shot or an intrauterine device (IUD).

Which method is best for you should be decided after you talk to your doctor. According to the National Institutes of Health (NIH), patches and pills can help relieve hot flashes, night sweats and vaginal dryness. Vaginal rings or creams are used for vaginal dryness and the ring may also help alleviate some urinary tract symptoms. Patches can deliver drugs that by-pass the first "pass" or metabolism through the liver which may lessen side effects; however, some women get irritation from the adhesives connected to patches.

Can hot flashes kill you?

No, hot flashes will not kill you. Though they may make you feel like you want to kill someone. Although often joked about, they can be a serious condition that adversely affects a women's quality of life. In many cases, hot flashes can interrupt sleep patterns which in turn can lead to irritability among other things. Sleep deprivation is also associated with more accidents which can be deadly so in a sense there could be a tangential relationship. There should be no jokes about hot flashes, but like I said, sometimes humor can help us get through the tough—and even hot—times in life. Stress reduction which could include finding reasons to laugh may be helpful.

Is it normal to forget things and lose part of your memory?

Memory loss is a common complaint among many women entering menopause. It is easy to assume that any memory change after the age of 40 could simply be a part of the natural aging process. One group of Boston researchers looked at it a different way. They posited that it was not a memory problem as much as a learning problem. You can't forget something you didn't know. At the core of the theory is the concept that their hectic lives and changing moods make it harder for women to keep track of daily occurrences.

According to an article in *Science Daily*, there is another change in thinking. It was originally understood that hormone therapy or MHT helped protect a women's memory if hormones are started soon as symptoms begin. Other studies have found that MHT could possibly increase the risk of developing dementia. Yet, another study found that there was no evidence that memory is affected by menopause. All these differing results add to the confusion that women and their doctors may share on this topic.

We all need a good night of sleep to retain memories. Hot flashes or night sweats could be related to impaired memory.

Do men go through menopause?

They do, in a way. At least there is a name for it—andropause. As men age, they experience a slow reduction in their production of testosterone. Unlike women; however, this is such a slow and steady process that symptoms are far less severe, if noticeable at all. Some men who reported symptoms include a reduction in libido, fatigue, depression, night sweats, and insomnia. There also hormone replacement therapy for men. Just as it isn't for women, this treatment should not be considered a silver bullet. There are risks, including a higher risk of prostate cancer. Others joke that the mid-life crisis when a man acquires a new fancy car and a new girlfriend or other toys to go with his new lifestyle may indicate that he is nearing or in andropause. However, there are no data to confirm it—just anecdotal reports.

When should I talk to my doctor about menopause?

As you start to go through perimenopause, it is important to talk about heart disease, osteoporosis, cancer and strokes. Framed in this discussion is whether you should consider hormone therapy. In the end, it is a personal decision and your doctor can give you the information you need to make the best decision for your health. You may want to talk to your doctor about whether you should continue to take oral contraceptives as well. You can still get pregnant even if your periods are irregular during this time. Contraceptives may help regulate your menstrual flow. If you do stay on them, though, it may be more difficult to know when you are going through menopause since there will only be some or no bleeding.

Keep in mind that discussions about menopause should not be a one time event. Find a doctor that you feel comfortable with discussing your most personal concerns and who is open to listening to you.

Can I take testosterone to increase my libido?

Research has shown that women who have low sexual desire after surgical menopause were helped by low doses of testosterone. One such study, however, noted that the influence of the hormone on mood and well-being requires further exploration. My feeling about women using testosterone is not to use it. A lot of women complain that their libido decreases during menopause and afterward. A post-menopausal ovary can still produce androgens or male hormones. We also get androgens from our adrenal glands. Some women want more, but there can be side effects including acne, beard growth, deepening of voice and male pattern baldness. There may also be an increased risk of heart disease and liver damage. Sometimes our libidos could be more dependent on our choice of partners.

Will my skin get wrinkled when I go through menopause?

There are estrogen receptors throughout the body, including the skin, brain and every organ. Some women notice that, after menopause, their skin appears more wrinkled. Estrogen is known to stimulate collagen renewal which can improve tone. With new cosmetic products and minimally invasive procedures, the need for estrogen for this effect is less relevant. Not smoking and staying out of the sun will also protect your skin to look more healthy and radiant.

CHAPTER FIVE
COSMIC COSMETOLOGY
—The Galaxy of Sex and Gender-based Medicine

"In those days spirits were brave,
the stakes were high, men were real men,
women were real women, and small furry
creatures from Alpha Centauri
were real small furry
creatures from Alpha Centauri."

—Douglas Adams
The Hitchhiker's Guide to the Galaxy

Every year, NASA would hold several video teleconferences on medical issues with the partners involved in the International Space Station. Many of the NASA field centers participate such as the Kennedy and Johnson Space Centers as well as the European and Russian Space Agencies. I always found the experience priceless. The information shared was valuable and, regardless of the few second delay, I picked up important visual cues from my colleagues by seeing them as they spoke.

One of the scientists from Moscow was in Washington, D.C. at NASA Headquarters to speak about the Russian space medicine program. Not too long before the meeting, he had given a speech at Moscow University. In his speech, he stated that women would not be the first space explorers to go to Mars. Instead, according to him, fragile women needed to be carried into space in the strong hands of men. My colleagues enjoyed that comment. They jokingly started calling me their fragile flower and offering to carry me in their strong hands around the office. I offered them catcher mitts with a smile.

As shocking as it sounds, his statement was not a surprise. Ironically, the Russians were the first to fly a woman into space in the 1960s. I thought about the scientist's earlier comments while he presented to the group. He spoke about Russian medical testing and countermeasures in space. At the end of his presentation, there was an opportunity for all of us to ask questions. I felt it was my duty to raise specific health issues facing women astronauts and cosmonauts.

"What specific countermeasures do you use to protect the health of woman in space?" I asked.

His answer was not unexpected. He said something about providing for the special reproductive needs of women. I think he was referring to menstruation. It was a start, no doubt, but I hoped for more.

Women's bodies respond differently to space travel. Women's cardiovascular and bone health need to be given sex-specific consideration. Instead, his response harkened back to the days of bikini medicine. We are now busy discussing our first steps to go to Mars. I think it was about time for a new paradigm.

While pondering the scientist's answer, he turned around looking at me and said, "Oh, yes, we also provide special face creams. Women still need to be women in space."

The camera was trained directly at me. I tried to keep my face frozen. I was amazed but did not want to show any reaction. It was tough.

Shortly after that comment, one of my colleagues made a wonderful remark. He was a respected doctor originally from Armenia. He looked me in the eye and said in his delightful accent:

"That brings a new meaning to the term Cosmic Cosmetology."

I laughed. The humor was important. It did not minimize the issue, but helped us to get past misconceptions and take a stand.

After the conference, I sent a light-hearted email message to NASA's Chief Medical Officer. In it, I suggested that instead of partnering with the National Institutes of Health, maybe we should start talks with Lancôme.

It was good for a laugh, but it also pointed out how far we were from honestly addressing sex and gender-based medicine. Misconceptions can be detrimental to our health. I'm not talking about who is better, stronger or smarter. I'm talking about recognizing similarities and differences between men and women so we can develop the most appropriate measures to keep everyone healthy in space and on Earth. We all deserve no less.

* * *

In January 2005, Lawrence Summers gave a talk at a conference entitled "Diversifying the Science and Engineering Workforce." At the time, he was the president of Harvard University. His speech addressed the underrepresentation of women in tenured science and engineering positions at research institutions. His comments implied that an innate difference between men and women may be the answer.

The audience was outraged. Nancy Hopkins, an MIT professor, walked out. As his words spread outside the walls of the conference, the reaction grew more hostile. In the end, his remarks contributed to him resigning his position at Harvard.

Some time later, Dr. Kathie Olsen, a former colleague at NASA, asked me to fill in for her at an American Association for the Advancement of Science conference. She was then the Associate Director at the White House Office of Science and Technology Policy. She was the Chief Scientist at NASA when I first met her. She was a strong proponent of sex and gender-based medicine.

I was asked to present on the impact of sex and gender on human adaptation to harsh environments. During the talk, I was asked about Dr. Summers' comments about women not excelling at math and science. At the time, he had just left Harvard.

The question made me think. Regardless of the harsh reaction, maybe he was not too far off. I do believe he missed a few cardinal points, but maybe it was a case of the messenger not the message. Lawrence Summers was known to be, at times, outspoken and gruff, but I can't say that his comment was totally out in left field. There are innate differences between men and women. That's why sex and gender-based medicine is so important.

I believe that women's brains are wired differently from men's. Let's use this analogy. Imagine two cars are lost in a city and both pull over for directions. One is driven by a man and the other by a woman. The man will probably ask for GPS coordinates and mileage while the woman will probably want landmarks, for example, "turn left at the blue house with white shutters." Both sexes get to the final destination, but the journey may not be the same.

Men and women definitely take in information differently. Not only that, we also use information differently. The system we live in; however, was created by a male-centric society—our founding fathers. Think about it. Ginger Rogers had to do everything backwards and in high heels.

Although I am half joking about Ginger Rogers, that kind of barrier permeates all our professions. So, maybe Lawrence Summers wasn't so far off. Maybe we need to accept that men and women process information differently and have to do it in an environment that is tailored to the male approach of learning.

When I gave the lecture at that scientific conference, I said the same thing about Dr. Summer's comments, but I didn't get a hostile response. There are times that women get lost in the process due to the system being constructed from a man's point of view. In a supportive environment, when we don't fight our innate abilities but embrace them, women can do just as well if not superior in some areas. Men can do better in some ways, too.

There is a physiological difference between the sexes. In most cases, our journeys are going to be different. We will get from point A to point B, but we might do it differently, and we should appreciate each other's path if we want to learn everything we can from our travels.

Although the messenger paid somewhat for the message, I think Dr. Summers did raise awareness. Increasing dialogue can be beneficial. For example, Harvard now has its first female president and committees designed to examine gender equity. Many universities across the nation are examining the issues to ensure that they recruit, retain and promote both men and women based on their abilities not because of or despite their gender. Perhaps, "we have a come a long way, baby" per an old tobacco slogan, and we still have many miles to go, but at least the journey has begun.

* * *

Let's start from the beginning. What is the difference between sex and gender? The Institute of Medicine (IOM) stated that when we examine "gender" differences, we are considering the psychosocial construct of individuals, how they regard themselves as male or female. When we examine "sex" perspectives, we are considering the biological aspects at the chromosomal or most basic biologic level.

In 2002, NASA joined with the University of Missouri to develop a conference that focused on sex and gender-based research. Our hope was that this conference would serve as a landmark event not only for NASA, but also for other agencies and organizations.

At the time, our goal was to review the current status of research on sex and gender-based differences in human adaptation to challenging environments. We also wanted to recommend research infrastructure and priorities so that we could eventually translate our findings into clinical care.

We selected six working groups that focused on the key systems of the body: musculoskeletal, cardiovascular, reproductive, neurological, immunological and behavioral.

Musculoskeletal Issues

Even though our astronauts use their muscles, they do not have the factor of gravity to maintain muscle mass just as we see with bone mass. Gravity is necessary to maintain muscle and bone mass. Over an extended time, such as a long-duration mission to Mars, this is extremely important. Significant loss in muscle mass was reported after only eleven days of spaceflight in data pooled from both sexes.

Obviously, sarcopenia—the rate of muscle loss—is a significant problem in space travel. We know that women have more slow-twitch muscle fibers, and men can have more fast-twitch muscle fibers. Whereas slow-twitch fibers are important for endurance, fast-twitch fibers give us a quick burst of energy. This is why we are probably not going to have the fastest woman ever beat the fastest man on this planet. Men aren't better than women, they're just constructed differently.

On Earth, we've observed that the rate of muscle loss in men parallel that in women, yet the detriment in muscle strength is greater in men. In space you tend to lose slow twitch fibers a lot more quickly than fast-twitch and some may be converted to fast twitch muscle fibers. This makes sense in that there is more of a need for quick bursts of energy rather than endurance in microgravity. So if women have slower twitch muscle fibers to begin with what will be the impact on muscle strength during spaceflight? Would there be less loss of strength compared to men?

NASA uses bed-rest data to simulate microgravity. For one week to three months, research subjects are put in a Trendelenburg position (i.e., subjects are laying flat in bed and their head tilted downward 30 to 40 degrees) which mimics being weightless.

Through these studies, we can assess the effects of immobilization on bone as well. On Earth we can generally lose about 1% of bone mass per year, but in space, it can be more than 1-3% per month. Bone quality could worsen as well. The risk of developing osteoporosis or significant bone loss or quality is a major concern for long duration space travel as it is on Earth especially as we age.

Most people consider osteoporosis a disease for women. In my opinion, that is a reversed bias. Look at the late Pope John Paul II. I believe he had osteoporosis. He had the tell tale stooped posture and he fractured his hip. For men, the disease is not always diagnosed. Many men don't ask their doctors about it. Doctors are often more focused on a man's prostate and his heart. Ironically, treating prostate cancer depletes hormones and can put a man at a higher risk for osteoporosis.

For me, it is a very personal issue. It is the disease that contributed to the passing of my mother. In fact, she was beating pancreatic cancer when she fell during the summer of 2009 and fractured her shoulder. This was after several falls and subsequent fractures to her wrists, arms and vertebrae impacting significantly the quality of her life. She developed pneumonia after she fractured her shoulder and died of an infection in the hospital. It is not so uncommon a story, but the true culprit is often overlooked.

As doctors, we sometimes overlook the bones because we don't see them nor do our patients. They are not obvious. Most of the time, osteoporosis does not reveal itself until a fracture occurs and than it can be too late.

When I was working for the government, I helped to create a national bone health campaign directed toward girls. People develop about 90 percent of bone mass by the age of 20, half of it during adolescence. Bone mass peaks in the mid 30s. From there, we slowly lose it, especially for women. Bone mass depletion accelerates to three to five percent a year after menopause for at least three to five years. Doctors do screen patients for bone lose. However, prevention is the best medicine.

With that in mind, we started the PowerfulBones/PowerfulGirls campaign. It was focused towards girls, aged 9-12, and their parents. We felt that this was the time period that girls establish behaviors that stay with them through their entire lives. It was important to educate them on bone health. We learned that young girls model their eating patterns after their mothers and use their fathers as role models for exercise. However, parents often don't know about bone building behaviors and so we needed to educate them as well.

Our idea was to keep it positive and focus on healthy behavior. Although substance abuse and eating disorders can have a negative impact on bone development, we stressed the importance of exercise, vitamin D and calcium. The research at the time showed that boys do well with calcium and exercise at that age. Think of the commercials you see on television all the time of boys drinking milk from the cartoon. They are also more likely to go to the gym at an earlier age to build their muscles.

The program was effective and is still on-going with a slightly different name. We may not see the impact of this campaign for years, but the hope is that it will significantly reduce women with osteoporosis and fractures as this generation ages.

The campaign got me thinking about my mother. She was lactose intolerant and did not drink milk and had been a smoker, both increasing her risk of getting the disease. Her diagnosis did not come about until she started to break her toes and ribs. When the doctor did a bone density study, she was found to have low bone mass especially in her spine. Maybe education earlier in life may have helped her avoid smoking. Smoking damages bone cells and increases the metabolism of estrogen which protects against bone loss. Maybe she could have found alternate ways to increase her calcium intake and her vitamin D. Later in life, I know I encouraged her to do all of that, but by then, the behaviors were set and the damage done. That's why educating yourself and your children are so important. You don't want to look back and ask, "What could I have done differently?"

My mother did stop smoking but the bone loss had occurred. Watching her made all of the family more aware of how important it is to take care of your body. We did not want to repeat what she had endured especially since osteoporosis has a strong genetic component. Every positive change in behavior can make a difference.

Our knowledge about the impact of space on sex differences in bone loss or osteopenia, the precursor to osteoporosis where bone density is lower than normal, is still limited quantitatively and qualitatively by the dEarth of studies in space and by the fact that the Trendelenburg test does not fully equate with microgravity. Thus, we have much to learn, especially in our understanding of what would be the best countermeasures to prevent or treat bone loss. For example, how effective is physical activity using resistance exercises with bungee cords and stationary bikes in space?

We can use hormonal therapy such as estrogen to prevent or treat osteoporosis on Earth. I remember discussing the possibility of prescribing sex hormones to astronauts. What will be the implications of hormone use in space for both men and women? We have no answers to these questions, but we do the best we can with what we have knowing that we may need to adapt it as the science evolves. It reminds me of the challenges we face when we try to practice sex and gender-specific medicine on Earth. Sometimes the data are not sufficient to address the possibly subtle but very real differences.

Most women know that osteoporosis is an elephant in the room for our health as we age. It causes the bones to become brittle. The name literally means "porous bones." It most commonly affects the wrist, hip or vertebrae. The National Osteoporosis Foundation estimates that 10 million Americans have osteoporosis and nearly 34 million suffer from low bone mass. Eighty percent of the 10 million are women. Pharmaceutical companies have targeted their advertising to women because of these numbers. Unfortunately, men are being missed and the consequences can be dire.

Just like heart disease, we should be cautious in labeling a disease by gender. Osteoporosis-related fractures in men result in considerable impairment, and the one year death rate after a hip fracture in men is twice that in women. This outcome could be attributable to the fact that osteoporosis is under-diagnosed and undertreated in men. Older men, especially those beyond the age of 65 years, need to undergo assessment for risk factors for osteoporosis too. The National Osteoporosis Foundation also recommends a bone mineral density test for men 70 years of age or older.

Cardiovascular Issues

Astronaut Shannon Lucid held the U.S. single-mission spaceflight endurance record for many years when she was on Russia's space station Mir in 1996. That record of 188 days, 4 hours, and 14 seconds was surpassed only a few years later. Her record for longest duration spaceflight was broken by fellow astronaut, Sunita Williams, crew of the International Space Station.

Shannon Lucid was truly a trailblazer. As a biochemist, she conducted a number of life science experiments while on Mir. She, along with other crew members, performed neuro-vestibular, cardiovascular, pulmonary, metabolic and musculoskeletal experiments on themselves. Their results would help NASA understand how the brain and nerves, the heart, lungs, hormones, muscle and bone adapted to the extreme environment of space.

We have found that many female astronauts returning from space travel experience orthostatic hypotension—dizzy spells. It is caused by a rapid fall in blood pressure. Interestingly, we also see this in small-frame male astronauts. We know that women have less tolerance to upright posture or gravitational stress than men have, primarily because of a reduced ability to maintain blood supply to the heart, but we don't know why. Is it an effect of the hormonal milieu? Does estrogen and testosterone contribute to this? We do know that women on Earth respond to cardiovascular stress with greater increased heart rates than men do, whereas men respond with greater increases in vascular resistance probably because of testosterone which causes blood vessels to constrict.

In July 2009, I was asked to serve on a panel at NASA evaluating medical standards for NASA pilots. I was the only woman on the panel. When the discussion turned to cardiovascular or heart disease, I found myself defending my thesis that heart disease is a medical concern for women who are even younger than what we would expect from our old beliefs about heart disease and that population is often considerably misdiagnosed.

When I was faced with questions from my colleagues on that panel, I quickly turned to the body of scientific evidence to refute what I considered a myth, that heart disease is a man's disease and only seen in women when they get older. I looked at the 2005-2006 National Health and Nutrition Examination Survey. It revealed that cardiovascular disease is the second leading cause of death among women ages 45-64 and the third leading cause of death in women ages 25-44. In 2008, the National Institutes of Health found that 17.1 per 100,000 women from ages 35-44, and 49.2 per 100,000 women from ages 45-54 had heart disease. That roughly translates to 35,000 women under the age of 55. It is not a small number.

Coronary heart disease is not just a man's disease. According to the American Heart Association, more women die annually from ischemic heart disease, characterized by reduced blood flow to the muscles of the heart, than men; and it is not just older women. The CDC has published data that states 38 percent of deaths among women are related to coronary heart disease, which is much higher than the rate for cancer. Although the fatality rate has gone down in recent history, it is still the leading cause of death in the United States and the rates have not gone down as significantly for women as compared to men.

Alarmingly, the advances we have seen in the field have not led to the kind of improvements for women that are there for men. Dr. Noel Bairey Merz among others conducted a review of the science behind why this has happened. They reviewed a large body of evidence on sex and gender-related differences pertaining to heart disease. One of their most disturbing findings suggests that the current means of early detection of the disease may not be as effective for women as it is for men. They suggest devising tests for women that look at patients with and without current symptoms such as chest pain.

The difference between men and women when it comes to heart attacks is very real. For example, 20 percent of women experience upper-abdominal pain, nausea and shortness of breath instead of the classic "elephant on the chest" sensation male patients identify. This may be one reason why many women have been sent home from the ER with an antacid and a prescription for an anti-anxiety drug.

As researchers have shown, it can be harder to diagnosis heart disease and heart attacks for women than it is for men. For example, traditional treadmill tests tend to be less accurate for women and an angiogram may not show plaques in their vessels since some women may have plaques in small vessels not visualized in an angiogram. Women, therefore, have to be their own best advocates. The first step, as always, is education and awareness. Knowledge of prevention and early signs of heart disease can lead to earlier intervention and longer, healthier lives.

Immunologic Issues

When we looked at immunology and space, a common thread appeared. No studies have been conducted to determine the effects of sex on the immune system in space. On Earth, we know that women are more susceptible to autoimmune diseases compared with men—approximately 80% occur in women. We also know that there is bone-marrow suppression during space travel. So, will resistance to infectious diseases be increased? What will be the impact of previous immunizations? What about cancer? Will there be relapses?

The immune system is so important in protecting the body against foreign "antigens" or invaders such as bacteria and viruses as well as to keep cells in our bodies from dividing uncontrollably leading to cancers. It is a complex dance between protection and repair and injury when the immune system can sometimes attack its own body leading to autoimmune diseases.

Back on Earth, when you think of immunology and sex, it is impossible not to address another pandemic—AIDS. It is generally understood that early in the course of the disease, women have been largely ignored in AIDS and HIV research. As would be expected, most early research focused more on pregnancy and childbirth than women suffering with the illness.

Let's look at some numbers. Researchers studied the differences in survival after an AIDS diagnosis between men and women. They found that women have a small but increasing mortality risk compared to men. Although factors such as race and age could influence the data, they found that sex and gender could not be ruled out.

According to the Henry Kaiser Family Foundation's 2007 data, 20 percent of the cumulative AIDS cases in the United States are women. Interestingly, the number increases to 26 percent when looking at new cases.

According to the United Nations Development Fund for Women, in 2006, women constituted half of the people living with AIDS worldwide. In sub-Saharan Africa, the percentage is a staggering 59 percent. So many children in Africa are without their mothers and even both parents leading to a generation of lost children. The tragedy of AIDS has cast a wide net across many generations. In their Executive Summary: Transforming the National AIDS Response, they outlined three "entry points for strengthening the gender equality and women's rights perspectives in the national AIDS coordinating authority." They include allocating resources to the understanding of the gender aspects of the disease worldwide, increasing gender-specific analysis, and ensuring that "women's voices are heard and count." I think these conclusions apply perfectly when looking at gender and medicine as a whole.

It is not just AIDS. According to a recent study in the *American Journal of Pathology*, eight percent of the population is affected by autoimmune diseases, and 78 percent of those affected are women. The exact cause of this discrepancy is not known. One thing we do know is that men and women's bodies react differently to infection. In women, we tend to see more antibodies; whereas in men, we see more inflammation. Antibodies are proteins in the blood that attempt to remove a virus or bacteria whereas inflammation is the body's vascular tissue response to harm. Although that response protects women more effectively against infection, it may also be part of the reason they develop more autoimmune diseases. But I also suspect that once a woman is infected, she mounts a very vigorous inflammatory response. This may cause more harm such as what is seen in a "cytokine storm" state where inflammatory cells are aggressively attacking the invader but can also cause tissue damage such as in the lungs and heart.

We also see differences in the incidence and location of cancer among men and women. For example, men are more likely to have bladder cancer than women. According to the American Cancer Society, of the 71,000 new cases in 2009, 52,800 were men.

It may not be as simple as that. Researchers have found that women are more likely to die of bladder cancer than men. A review of the research found that women are 80-114% more likely to die of bladder cancer in the first year following diagnosis. Another study looked into whether this has something to do with the stage of the disease at diagnosis. It would make sense that if the disease was not diagnosed until later, that the prognosis would be worse. What they found was surprising. It is unlikely that time of diagnosis was the real culprit. Much more needs to be explored.

Lung cancer has its own unique sex differential. Scientists have found that, although the rate of occurrence of lung disease in men has leveled off, it is still rising in women. Researchers that went through the current data available found some interesting things. Women who have never smoked are more likely to get lung cancer than men that have never smoked. They concluded that the increasing rate found in women cannot be explained by exposure to cigarette smoke, smoking history or body size. They posit that women have a higher susceptibility to tobacco carcinogens than men.

Clearly, having a greater understanding of sex differences in cancer can impact how one is diagnosed and treated. For example, women may also respond better to chemotherapy for lung cancer compared to men.

Neurological Issues

NASA investigated the impact of space on the neuro-vestibular system including John Glenn's spaceflight on the Discovery in 1998 and the Spacelab mission called NeuroLab. NeuroLab investigated how the nervous system responds to the challenges of spaceflight. Experiments have shown that when astronauts first travel into space, both men and women can experience space sickness. Their eyes and ears fail to sync up. Their eyes may say that they are facing forward but their otolith organs, the sensory cells in the ears, tell them they are falling back to Earth. Within three or four days, equilibrium is generally reestablished.

Many astronauts feel space sickness or nausea during this early period. Although there are countermeasures to alleviate space sickness, it can still be an important problem. For example, what if an astronaut feels ill during a crisis? We also know from studies on Earth that women present with symptoms of imbalance and disequilibrium twice as frequently compared to men. Women are also at a higher risk for motion sickness, and certainly morning sickness is a very common problem in pregnancy. I think this is an interesting area to explore to see if men and women are impacted differently while in space.

NASA takes any neuro-vestibular interruption seriously because there is no accident forgiveness in the harsh environment of space. In their review of the existing science, NASA scientists found that the number of women astronauts studied prior to their research was too small, and the other factors affecting neuro-vestibular function too great, to come to a valid conclusion about gender or sex-specific differences. But time and experience will tell.

People always say that, neurologically, boys and girls develop differently. In my house, it was obvious. I have a twin brother. My mom told me that I walked several months earlier. My brother would try to trip me up so I would crawl with him. I was also a nonstop talker. I have to believe that our predictable differences were related to the difference in wiring between men and women.

The point of John Gray's immensely popular book, *Men Are From Mars And Women Are From Venus*, was that men and women communicate differently. From men being withdrawn while dealing with stress, to women needing to talk things through. He discussed many of the stereotypical male/female behaviors people talk about every day. But how true are they?

Response to that book ranged from total agreement to downright anger. Experts don't always agree either. One study looked at nonverbal communication. They rated how men and women performed twenty behaviors linked to body language. They found women to be better at sending and understanding the message through body language. Men, on the other hand, were found to be louder and to perform more actions that were not considered to mean anything. Interestingly, the ratings backed up the findings of the study, showing that our beliefs about body language were accurate.

Another study found there to be little difference between the manner in which men and women communicate. An assistant professor at Purdue University found the concept of the book not only wrong but possibly harmful. Through interviews and questionnaires she collected data from both men and women. It showed that men and women communicate very similarly when it came to friendships, taking advice and the processing of "comforting comments."

From my experience, and considering the volumes upon volumes of work dissecting communications between the sexes, I feel there must be some genetic and evolutionary differences to the way male and female brains work. When I say that, I tend to get laughs from my audience which is not my intention. Think about it. Back in the Neanderthal days, women needed to raise children and make sure there was a fire. In doing that, they had to bond with the other women in the clan. This is described as a "tend and befriend" response. Men were out hunting together. During stressful times, they may be more likely to "fight or flight" such as retreating into that cave. They needed more directional thinking, focusing only on the goal at hand, while women needed to be proficient at multi-tasking. Maybe that is why women's corpus callosum, the neural pathway between the right and left sides of the brain, have been found to be more active, thus women tend to be better at using both sides of their brain. It's evolutionary thinking, and not everyone wants to hear it.

A few years ago, a study of the brain done by the University of California found something very interesting. Looking at scans of the brain, they learned men and women's brains are, in fact, different. According to their findings, men have about six-and-a-half times more gray matter than women. Women, however, have ten times as much white matter. What I find most intriguing is that gray matter is generally associated with the part of the brain that processes information and white matter deals with the connections between those processing centers. When you stop and think, the processing part of the brain is useful for subjects like math. The networking part of the brain is good for language. In the end, the study found no difference in intelligence associated with the physiological differences they observed. It does make me wonder. Did this study partially support what Lawrence Summers suggested about the sexes?

Genitourinary Issues

In terms of reproductive health, there is very little data on sex-based differences in reproductive biology that are relevant to spaceflight. We do know radiation exposure is extremely important. We are particularly concerned with germ cells also known as eggs or sperm and carcinogenesis, the process of normal cells mutating into cancer. We previously thought radiation exposure was just a concern for women requiring protection of the ovaries, but we now know that sperm cells are also very sensitive to radiation damage. Thus, we need to focus on the reproductive health of male astronauts as well.

Reproductive issues related to spaceflight are topics that many find interesting. I am frequently asked, "Is there sex in space?"

Audiences often think I am going to discuss something else when I talk about sex, but I am referring to its impact on how we adapt to space. Studies have shown that men's testosterone levels can drop during long-term stays in the isolated research stations of Antarctica. As soon as you introduce a woman, their testosterone levels rise dramatically and men even experience increased beard growth. This observation is truly fascinating and has significant implications for space travel.

Many health issues affecting the urinary tract affect men and women differently. Kidney stones, hard deposits of salt and minerals found in the kidney, are more common in men. This could be related to the differences in the pH or acidity of the urine leading to more stone formation in men. According to the National Institutes of Health data from 1988-1994, 6.3 percent of men have them while only 4.1 percent of women. When it comes to urinary tract infections, the numbers go the other way. Again in 1994, 13.3 percent of women had a urinary tract infection compared to only 2.3 percent of men. This may because the urethra is so close to vagina and the anus and bacteria can be transported to the urethra from sexual intercourse or wiping after a bowel movement. Astronauts have had kidney stones and urinary tract infections in space which can be quite painful and can impact a mission as it does our lives on Earth although treatments for these conditions in space are more limited.

Urination is another area of interest. I think the whole concept of men and women using the bathroom in zero-g add a dimension of novelty. Also, people's imaginations are quite vivid.

I remember going on a tour of the space shuttle simulator at Johnson Space Center. As we neared the lavatory, our guide told us that astronauts have to complete training in how to use the facilities prior to launch, a form of potty training. When we got there, all of us on the tour immediately noticed a camera in the toilet with a monitor on the wall. This led to the most interesting discussion of the trip. In the end, we realized that the live feed was to ensure proper position. Although you can imagine how serious an issue it is to astronauts in space, on land it is still the stuff of middle school humor.

The bathroom isn't the only aspect of space travel where men and women differ, but it does create some issues for astronauts. Whether the challenges of using the facilities have anything to do with it, men and women both tend to eat and drink less in space. This can lead to dehydration and weight loss which can also impact how astronauts metabolize drugs.

In relation, the body's ability to absorb medication changes in space. We've already seen on Earth how men and women metabolize drugs differently. Back in 2001, the General Accounting Office (GAO) looked at 10 drugs that the FDA forced off the market during the previous four years. It was found that eight of the ten drugs removed from the market represented higher risks for women than men.

It is clear from the government's findings that drugs affect men and women differently. Irritable bowel syndrome is a perfect example. A medication to treat this disease is Lubiprostone. Interestingly, the FDA has only approved this drug for women. So next time you get a prescription, ask your doctor and your pharmacist if the medication has been tested on men and women. Most likely they will not know the answer, but it will make more them think about it.

Behavioral Health Issues

It has not been observed that significant gender differences exist in the psychosocial factors important for long-duration spaceflight. Yet, some of the factors examined have interesting implications on Earth.

One factor was gender reaction to isolation and life-threatening risk conditions with limited possibilities for rescue. Interestingly, some terrestrial or Earth-based studies have shown a significant gender difference in surviving disasters. Scientists found that a disaster lowers the life expectancy of women more than it does men. Data showed that the stronger the disaster, the bigger the impact. Because women's life expectancies are higher in normal scenarios, disasters actually reduce the gender gap.

They also found that certain groups were more vulnerable to the impact of a disaster. They felt, however, that physiological factors between sexes were not the most contributing factor. Issues such as previous exposure to trauma and inequitable access to resources also played a role. Their research found that it was "socially constructed gender-specific vulnerability of females built into everyday socioeconomic patters that lead to the relatively higher female disaster mortality rates compared to men." This finding may explain why similar findings were not reached when looked at female astronauts, a more homogenous group with similar social constructs and resources as their male counterparts.

People have different opinions of the perfect group dynamic. Some researchers found that a team's perception of itself can vary from what an outside observer thinks of their performance, particularly in mixed gender and race groups. Researchers performed an experiment that looked at groups that were homogenous and groups that varied with respect to gender and race. The heterogeneous group assessed their team's effectiveness lower than the homogenous group did. Ratings from outside sources; however, showed no difference in effectiveness between the groups.

Lastly, the challenge of limited privacy and the constant interpersonal contact and confinement of space travel is a critical issue. Privacy is an important issue even on Earth. Walk outside, especially in urban areas, and look up. I can almost guarantee you will see a video camera pointing down on you. I once met a friend in Times Square and we sat down to talk and noticed a sign that said the area was under video surveillance. We were sharing emotional experiences relating to the recent illnesses and deaths in our families. I could only imagine what the observers on the other end thought when they saw the pained expressions on our faces.

A study looked at this phenomenon of the digital age and how it relates to gender. They surveyed 120 people who had just walked across a plaza and were unknowingly videotaped. Although they found most people "upheld some modicum of privacy in public," more women expressed concerned about being watched. Cyber stalking is a real issue that garnered legislation in California as far back as 1999. It was also addressed in the Violence Against Women Act of 2000. Just think about what ESPN reporter Erin Andrews went through when she was unknowingly videotaped in a hotel room and the video was leaked online. This behavior is becoming another form of violence against women.

Mental health issues, like other health concerns, have gender specific connections on Earth that can't be ignored. According to the CDC data on suicide rates in the US from 1990 to 2004, boys, ages 10 to 14 were almost twice as likely to commit suicide compared to girls. At the age of 15 to 19, they were more than three times as likely; from 20 to 24 almost five times. On top of that, boys were even more likely to make an attempt with a firearm. Obviously this data must be considered by mental health professionals when trying to prevent suicide.

Substance abuse is another mental health issue that follows the same history as most health issues in how they are examined from a gender-based perspective. The National Institute on Drug Abuse focused gender-specific studies on how drugs affected pregnancy, maternal health and child development. The focus on women related to their reproductive status and care-giving capacity. Finally, during the last decade, their policy changed and they started to look into the general causes and consequences of female drug abuse.

By refocusing their research, the Institute found gender differences in how women start using drugs, how their addiction grows and how they quit. They found that women may be more sensitive to the "reward" aspect of addiction. They also found that the menstrual cycle may also affect the intensity of drug's affect.

In 2004, I went to Antarctica on a former Russian research vessel. When I was getting ready to leave, I was asked to have a physical. At the time, I noticed that they did not ask for a psychological evaluation. I found that to be perplexing. We were going into one of the harshest climates on the planet and good psychological health and adaptability was essential. It did not make sense that this was not examined.

We set sail with forty individuals and a Russian crew. We got to the Antarctic and started the adventure of a lifetime. Some explorers did under ice diving and kayaked with whales. Others, such as myself, hiked the barren landscape and surveyed the pristine beauty from small zodiac boats.

Within a week, one woman on the trip emotionally decompensated. She had a psychotic breakdown and was no longer allowed to dive under the ice. In response, she threatened to slash the Zodiacs, the inflatable boats we used to leave the ship. I think she wanted us all to suffer like she was.

Eventually, the Captain had her quarantined to her room. We were all dependent on each other for safety. As her threat showed, a very unstable person with is put us all at risk even more than a physical ailment may have.

On a day following her quarantine, I took a motion sickness drug and got sleepy. I missed the Captain calling for an all-hands meeting. When I woke up, it was a bizarre scene. I wondered around the ship but didn't see anyone. I climbed up to the bridge and found the "Otto Pilot," a blown up penguin balloon, named Otto, behind the wheel. I heard something below and followed the sound to the small classroom on the lower level of the ice cutter. When I peeked in, I found the woman who had been quarantined now watching diving videos.

I felt like I had walked into a horror movie. In a moment of confusion, from my medication, all I could think was that she had killed the crew and that I was the only one left. Eventually, I found everyone in the lounge that had been accidentally locked, but the moment stuck with me. The crew had under-estimated what this woman would do and that she could escape from her room. They did not take her illness seriously. She was in need of care and close observation. All too often, women's needs are ignored or minimized especially in the realm of mental health.

Gender differences in mental health are striking. Twice as many women are likely to have affective disorders such as depression but unfortunately, only a quarter are diagnosed and of that group, only a quarter are effectively treated.

* * *

Gender equality in science is one of the most important aspects of ensuring everyone receives the best healthcare they deserve. During the 1990s, the federal government began to address these concerns. In 1993, the National Institutes of Health (NIH) Revitalization Act was signed into law, requiring the inclusion of women in all clinical research and analysis of results by sex for phase 3 clinical trials. The US Food and Drug Administration also published guidelines in 1993 for evaluating the influence of sex on drug metabolism which encouraged the inclusion of women in safety and dosing studies.

Although a 2001 follow-up audit by the General Accounting Office (GAO) found that women are now enrolled in NIH-funded clinical trials at appropriate representational rates, substantial deficits remained.

In 2008, I went to a space medicine summit. It is held every May at Rice University and brings together scientists and doctors from all across the world to discuss the latest in space medicine. People come from all over the globe including China, Russia, and Europe.

On the first day, there was a presentation by a panel about what we need to do to prepare astronauts for long duration space travel. At the end, I stood up to ask a question. I wondered what the ideal crew composition should be. A Russian scientist on the panel said it would be an all male crew. I couldn't resist, so I wryly added that some studies show women work well collaboratively. Maybe there should be an all female crew.

Later, when the sessions had ended and we all attended the reception, the Russian scientist approached me with his translator. We sat down and had a great conversation. We talked through the merits of a mixed gender crew—the advantages and disadvantages, and what men and women could learn from each other. The room we were in, the

Baker Institute at Rice University was filled with people talking and laughing. We sat at a large round table as people milled and mingled around us. I hardly noticed because I was so engrossed in the conversation.

We had to speak through a translator who was a woman. I remember watching her facial expressions and thinking that she had a vested interest in the conversation. She was so good that we never missed a beat. My off-the-cuff attempt at humor during the summit had opened the door to one of the most frank and useful gender discussions of my career.

Old myths die hard. As we prepare to travel to the Moon, Mars or even asteroids, it is imperative that medicine catches up. We have to break down stereotypes. In fact, the space program is a great catalyst. In space, the stakes are higher and the dynamic is fast and perilous. What better place can there be for us to bypass the simplicity of old-fashioned views of gender and sex and finally sit down, or float in zero-g for that matter, and learn from each other?

When I think about the very real possibility that a woman will one day step foot on Mars, I hope that, by then, we'll make sure that her entire body is as healthy as possible in space and on Earth. Women and men deserve equal healthcare tailored to their individual needs.

* * *

Prior to the end of the last century, it was generally understood that the science of medicine did not adequately research the differences in health between men and women. Most studies, except possibly early research on osteoporosis and pregnancy, used white men as their subjects. A woman was essentially considered a small man, "but with a uterus." When the male-centric nature of healthcare began its metamorphosis, the early advances were not exactly what we needed. Women's clinics painted the walls of their exam rooms pink in an effort to attract and address the needs of their patients.

Eventually, science got it right. Researchers began to study the differences between men and women and the findings were astounding. So much has been discovered with more to come, and those discoveries will improve and save lives.

Stellar Questions:

Are there sex differences in diabetes?

Diabetes is one condition for which sex differences have increasingly been investigated. Acute complications do vary between men and women. Although earlier in the 20th century, more women were diagnosed with Type II diabetes, a study found it to be equally prevalent now. This may be related to the growing obesity epidemic in the nation for both men and women. Gestational diabetes increases a woman's risk to develop diabetes after the pregnancy.

Recently, scientists have been researching the role of testosterone in diabetes. One study followed a population of men over years and evaluated their hormone levels. They found that low total testosterone predicted the development of diabetes. This finding could help develop an early warning system for men.

Why do thyroid disorders seem to affect more women than men?

Some thyroid disorders, including Hashimoto thyroiditis (hypothyroidism) and Graves' disease (hyperthyroidism), are seven to 10 times more prevalent in women than in men. This finding may be related to the increased predilection of women for autoimmune diseases. There is a tendency for these diseases to manifest during major hormonal shifts during puberty, pregnancy, and menopause. Diagnosis and treatment of thyroid diseases during pregnancy are a unique concern. For example, the overall prevalence of post-partum thyroid dysfunction is four percent; however, the prevalence is approximately 20 percent in women with Type 1 diabetes.

In men, thyroid diseases tend to occur at a later age than in women and to be more severe. A 2000 statement by the American Thyroid Association recommends that all adults undergo measurement of their serum thyroid stimulating hormone, TSH, concentration beginning at age 35 years and every five years thereafter.

Is aspirin effective to protect against heart disease in women?

Aspirin has been used to combat heart disease for almost forty years. It can decrease the pain associated with the disease and inhibit the formation of blood clots. One popular study, the Women's Health Study, looked at how effective aspirin is for female patients. The researchers conducted a ten-year study on the usage of low-dose aspirin and found it did not prevent first heart attacks in women, but it did help prevent strokes. Women 65 years or older saw the greatest benefit from taking aspirin. They did see a reduced risk of heart attack. However, men did not have stroke protection, only heart attack protection at all ages when they took aspirin. Women and men are at risk for gastro-intestinal bleeding with aspirin.

Are Attention Deficit Hyperactivity Disorder and Autism more common in boys?

Attention Deficit Hyperactivity Disorder might be the most commonly diagnosed disorder for children. The symptoms include difficulty focusing and controlling behavior. According to CDC data, boys are more likely than girls to be diagnosed, 9.5 percent compared to 5.9 percent.

Autism is a developmental disorder that causes the brain of sufferers to filter information differently. It can cause serious communication and behavioral issues. Again according to CDC data, boys are four to seven times more likely to be diagnosed than girls. Studies are also beginning to show that although the age of the father is an important risk factor, the risk increases more with mothers who are over the age of 40.

Why do women live longer than men?

There are a many theories about why women live longer than men. According to one study, the answer is in the menstrual cycle. They posited that estradiol, a hormone released during menstruation increases heart rate by 20 percent, in essence acting as a regular source of intense exercise.

Others have suggested more social and environmental reasons. Some think it is because men are far more likely to participate in high-risk behavior. Others cite the fact that women tend to suffer from cardiovascular disease at an older age. Still others claim life's stresses are the reason.

One thing is for sure. The life of a woman has changed drastically over the past century. It will be interesting to see how changing family dynamics and increasing professional opportunities for women will affect these statistics.

CHAPTER SIX
A NATION OF GHOSTS
—The Invisible Injuries of War

"Never, never, never believe any war will be smooth and easy, or that anyone who embarks on the strange voyage can measure the tides and hurricanes he will encounter. The statesman who yields to war fever must realize that once the signal is given, he is no longer the master of policy but the slave to unforeseeable and uncontrollable events."

—Sir Winston Churchill

On October 26, 2009, the Theater of War came to Washington, D.C. at the Shakespeare Theater. This event was sponsored by the Department of Veterans Affairs and the Department of Defense as part of their Mental Health Summit. I was invited to participate on the panel as a member of the Blue Star Families, a bi-partisan organization formed by military families to support military family issues. During 2009, the Theater of War presented readings of Sophocles' Ajax and Philoctetes to military communities.

Bryan Doerries was the translator and director of this performance. He stated that, "These ancient plays timelessly and universally depict the psychological and physical wounds inflicted upon warriors by war." It is his hope that by presenting these plays, "it will demystify and de-stigmatize psychological injury and to facilitate open dialogue with members of the military family." The panel that follows the reading serves an important purpose. It is a frank discussion about the challenges that service members, their families, and those who care for them face each day.

Bryan Doerries told me that he has performed this play to audiences on military bases, hospitals, homeless shelters, and theaters. Generally, the audience participates by sharing their experiences with the panel. It was suggested that Greek drama was a form of story telling and a tool for therapy for veterans thousands of years ago. It is a creative method to help the audience feel safe and comfortable about sharing their personal journeys. One could consider it a form of group therapy.

Ajax tells the story of a warrior who becomes depressed near the end of the Trojan War. He attempts to murder his commanding officers but fails and eventually commits suicide. Philoctetes is the story of a Greek warrior who is marooned on a deserted island after sustaining an injury. Both tales reveal poignant aspects to the trauma of war and its impact on family and fellow troops. The actors in the readings included Adam Driver, Terrence Howard, Elizabeth Marvel, and David Strathairn. They all performed superbly. It was a simple set—a table with microphones and no costumes. Their emotion and turmoil were reflected in their voice inflections and movements of their heads and eyes. We all sat transfixed throughout the readings.

I sat in the front row with other members of the panel which included two members of the military, a doctor from the Uniformed Services, and a chaplain. Each provided their own reflections of how the war impacted their lives. Sitting on the panel from center stage, I could see several generals sitting in the front row with many seats taken in the auditorium by other members of the military and participants from the Mental Health Summit. We each had a few minutes to speak followed by questions from the audience.

I had a chance to share my experience as a member of the military family who has faced the challenges of a loved one coming back from war. I must admit that it was easier to do a formal medical presentation as a doctor, but I felt that it was important to share and connect with others who faced similar situations. As we know, feeling isolated and alone in our journeys can be difficult. I could see many heads nod while I spoke, which indicated to me that I was perhaps a voice for those who could not speak. Yet, I also felt that I had to be careful to not say anything that could potentially damage a military career or cause pain or embarrassment for the family.

I often use the expression "loved one" rather than identify my family member in the military in order to protect privacy. I have faced the challenges that other families have probably also endured and that is some service members don't want to or are unable to because of their injuries to accept that changes or problems have occurred. Perhaps, they are afraid that their careers will be ruined or that they will be considered weak. It is also tragic when the injuries have affected self awareness and cognition to the point where they are not even aware that they are hurting themselves and others. As with any illness, if one does not own it, treatment cannot be administered. Heartbreak ensues for everyone involved. My situation was compounded by the poor care that was administered which led to more damage being done to the point where there was no longer any ability to acknowledge that there was a problem. All I could do was put out fires and try to keep the doors open for help—a hopeless task.

We have made some progress taking care of our wounded warriors, but the miles ahead are still significant. Changing ignorance or disbelief or denial would take more than a theater production or the monologue of a woman who has witnessed changes in her family member and faced the difficulties of trying to find medical care. I knew that if I had experienced the suffering and anguish of losing a loved one in front of my eyes, and, I as a doctor could not navigate through the medical system, I was not optimistic that others could do better. I wanted the military brass to know that. Yes, progress has been made, but we are not where we need to be—yet.

HARD BLOWS

One of the most troubling injuries in war is head trauma. The public understands the complexity of this type of injury with the death of Natasha Richardson in 2009. Although a civilian, Natasha Richardson's death shocked the world and her experience can shed light on what happens to soldiers who have head injuries. Apparently, Ms. Richardson experienced an unexceptional tumble on the beginner ski slopes, yet she died from a significant bleed in her brain. As a doctor who has seen this all too often in the emergency room, my initial reaction to reports of her accident was that the news would not be good.

I first witnessed this sort of tragedy when I was an intern in San Francisco General Hospital. A college student had fallen off his scooter and came to the emergency room with a small cut over his eyebrow. He indicated that he wasn't wearing a helmet at the time of the fall, but was only going a few miles an hour down the street when his scooter hit a small rock. During the evaluation, he answered my questions reasonably and calmly. He denied having a headache, blurred vision, or nausea. As I began to stitch the cut, he started to become agitated - shouting out math formulas before becoming unresponsive.

Clearly something major was happening. I took a look into his eyes and noticed that one of his pupils was growing larger than the other. This is known as "blowing a pupil" and indicated massive brain injury. I knew it was possible that there was so much pressure in his skull from bleeding that his brain might begin to herniate out the base of his skull through an area called the foramen magnum. Immediately, I called the neurosurgery team. A CT scan showed that he had developed an epidural hematoma, which is basically a giant bruise on the outer surface of the brain beneath the skull. Luckily he survived, but it was only because he had immediate access to brain surgery to relieve the building pressure.

Fortunately, many of the small bumps that we take on the head do not have disastrous consequences. Our skulls can protect us. Sometimes, though, the force of the impact against the skull can cause a bruise and bleeding to occur. We used to think that our brains could handle these tiny hemorrhages—often without horrible repercussions—but now we are reassessing that assumption. New studies evaluating football players show that there can be delayed effects from head traumas that occurred months or even years before any visible symptoms. Early forms of dementia with memory loss, mood and personality changes, and cognitive or thinking deficits are associated with these injuries.

I am very concerned about our military population and their vulnerability to head injuries. A Rand report from 2008 found that over 300,000 troops suffer from traumatic brain injury. I have to think the numbers are much higher than that. So many service members don't report that they've been hurt. Others don't realize that the vibration from a grenade explosion or gun firing can cause small hemorrhages or bleeds in the brain. If someone has experienced any hearing deficit from combat, you can be sure that there has been an impact on his or her neurological system and care should be taken to evaluate the potential impact on the brain.

There are now some new functional magnetic resonance imaging (fMRI) machines that help detect small bleeds, but many are missed on the usual imaging devices. The University of Pittsburg is evaluating the use of imaging machines that use high tesla or powerful magnets to detect injuries in the brain.

I am also worried that even psychological changes in troops may not appear immediately after small head traumas, making it difficult to connect the two incidents. How many cases of post-traumatic stress disorder (PTSD) are actually due to traumatic brain injury (TBI), which has been missed or ignored and now manifests as psychological impairment? What are the long-term consequences of not treating these injuries at the time they occur? How would we best treat them? Some studies are showing that we need to diagnose immediately even on the battlefield so that troops get medical care quickly which can improve outcomes.

In 2007, the Veteran's Administration (VA) implemented a computer-based screening process to identify patients with mild TBI. A GAO report from 2008 identified some of the challenges faced by the VA. They included a lack of existing diagnostic tools and that many symptoms of TBI are similar to PTSD. The VA outlines a number of things a patient can do with TBI to help recovery. They include not overexerting, returning to normal day-to-day activities, and avoiding alcohol.

When treating TBI, often the process is case-by-case depending on the seriousness of the damage to the brain. In an article from the *New England Journal of Medicine*, Susan Okie, M.D. looked at the case of a veteran, David Emme. He endured a brain injury from an explosion in Iraq. According to Emme, after the injury, he had to "learn what things were again." He "knew what they were—just didn't know what the names were."

His speech and language therapist, Laura Battiata, reported that Emme's speech was "nonsensical" when evaluated ten days after the injury. His treatment involved work on "deductive-reasoning tasks," and "basic problem—solving tasks." In many cases, treatment must delve down to the basics of functioning on a day-to-day basis. That is why TBI is such a huge challenge facing so many veterans of Iraq and Afghanistan.

Quoted in the article, Deborah Warden, a neurologist at Walter Reed Medical Center, commented on the Joint Theater Trauma Registry's findings that 22 percent of injured soldiers treated at a medical center in Germany had sustained wounds to the head, face and neck. Warden said that the proportion for the two wars is probably higher than that. Kevlar armor and helmets are one reason for the high numbers. It has improved survival rates by shielding the body and helmets have reduced the number of penetrating head wounds. Yet, they cannot protect all of the face, neck and head and cannot stop "closed brain injuries."

Most adults with mild TBI recover completely. With moderate and severe TBIs, however, there are often lingering effects. Clearly, due to the nature of the wars in Iraq and Afghanistan, TBI is a significant issue facing veterans. Treating it can be a challenge due to the complexity of the injuries and the array of symptoms for each case. Not to mention that these injuries are happening in high stress situations.

A study done in August, 2009 reiterated the tie between TBI and PTSD. Researchers looked at 94 veterans who were screened with the VA's traumatic brain injury screening program and found to show signs of TBI. They found that veterans who screened positive for mild TBI also had high rates of PTSD. It suggested, however, that the screening process might not differentiate between PTSD and TBI because they are "defined, in part, by the same events and the same self-reported symptoms. The study suggests that "interdisciplinary rehabilitation teams need to include mental health professionals with expertise in PTSD" when treating veterans with TBI.

POST-TRAUMATIC STRESS DISORDER

According to Glenn Schiraldi's book, *The Post-Traumatic Stress Disorder Sourcebook*, post-traumatic stress disorder (PTSD) is characterized as "extreme general arousal and/or arousal following exposure to internal or external triggers." Signs of arousal include trouble sleeping, irritability, hyper-vigilance and an exaggerated startle reflex.

The VA defines PTSD as "an anxiety disorder that can occur after you have been through a traumatic event." They outline four different types of symptoms to the disorder: 1) reliving the event, 2) avoiding situations that remind you of the event, 3) feeling numb, and 4) feeling keyed up. Along with experiencing symptoms, a sufferer may be more likely to have drinking or drug problems, feel depressed, have employment and relationship problems, or experience other physical symptoms.

The treatments outlined by the VA include cognitive behavioral therapy, eye movement desensitization and reprocessing, and medications such as selective serotonin reuptake inhibitors. In cognitive therapy, a therapist tries to get the patient to change the way he or she thinks about the trauma they survived. They help identify the thoughts that stimulate extreme reactions and find more accurate ways to process them. One of the biggest challenges is often convincing the patient they were not at fault for the traumatic event.

Eye movement desensitization and reprocessing is similar to cognitive therapy in that it attempts to help the patient change the way he or she reacts to their memories of trauma. While the patient recounts troubling memories, the therapist may move his or her hand in front of the patient's face, and the patient is supposed to focus on the movement, distracting the mind. Selective serotonin reuptake inhibitors are antidepressants. They include medications such as Prozac and Zoloft. Each raises the level of serotonin in the patient's brain. Serotonin is a neurotransmitter that plays a role in regulating mood, sleep and appetite.

Some studies have evaluated the role that morphine can play to decrease the incidence of PTSD. Researchers looked at almost 700 injured soldiers. Of that number, 243 were diagnosed with PTSD and 453 were not. They then looked at whether morphine was used in "early resuscitation and trauma care." Among the PTSD patients, they found that 61 percent received morphine; and among the non-PTSD patients, 76 percent received morphine. They concluded that the use of morphine may reduce the risk of developing PTSD after injury.

In an editorial relating to this study, Matthew J. Friedman, M.D., Ph.D., Executive Director of the National Center for Posttraumatic Stress Disorder, asked about the use of morphine in soldiers who are not severely injured. The idea of giving everyone morphine after a stressful situation may not be realistic. Holbrook's research, however, brings up the possibility of there being what Dr. Friedman refers to as a "morning-after pill." He assumes that PTSD is caused by Pavlovian fear conditioning— "the adrenergic activation of the amygdale during the trauma event facilitates encoding of traumatic memories" which means that chemical messengers stimulate a part of the brain that is important for emotional processing. As such, a response has been blocked in lab experiments with rats using propranolol—a beta blocker used mainly for hypertension or high blood pressure as well as to decrease the stress response such as fast heart beats and anxiety. Dr. Friedman stresses that more thought should be put into the use of such chemicals as a possible "morning-after pill" to prevent PTSD.

In 2009, I had an opportunity to present to Congress my thoughts on the "invisible wounds" of war. According to a 2008 RAND report, nearly 20% of veterans who have returned from Iraq and Afghanistan suffer from PTSD or major depression. I think that these numbers are actually low, since the report was based on extrapolated data from a survey of less than 2,000 troops. We now know that the number of Army suicides increased for years after the Iraq War began, and this was the first time since the Vietnam War that the Army suicide rate surpassed the civilian suicide rate.

I found that I could not speak about what was occurring in my life to others especially those who were not associated with the military. It was not because people did not care but more because they just did not understand. At the beginning of both wars, no one was talking about traumatic brain injury or post-traumatic stress disorders. In fact, there were even doctors who did not believe that PTSD or mild TBI actually existed. Some troops could not get disability as it was hard to prove. Physical injuries which could be seen had a greater chance of being compensated.

I could no longer be silent. Even if I could not immediately help my own family at least I could try to make a difference for others. In June 2009, there was a hearing on improving mental healthcare screening and care for troops pre- and post-deployment. The bill under discussion was the Post Deployment Assessment Act of 2009. It required live mental health screenings for soldiers deployed to combat.

The Senate hearing room, with its elegant wood paneling and high ceilings, was filled to the brim and every seat was taken. People were even standing near the windows and out in the doorway. I was seated in the middle of a very long table and was flanked by two colonels: Colonel Jeff Ireland, Director of the Montana National Guard, and Colonel Peter Duffy (retired), Deputy Director of the National Guard Association. We were joined by three others including two psychologists and Mr. Patrick Campbell, Chief Legislative Counsel for Iraq and Afghanistan Veterans of America. Mr. Campbell shared his experiences of how difficult it was to get mental healthcare while on active duty and how he was inappropriately questioned about his symptoms and needs when he returned home to the U.S.

During the briefing, staffers took copious notes and the audience remained completely silent. I don't think I've ever spoken to a more attentive group of people. I usually don't like to use prepared remarks, but we had tight time limits and I wanted to be sure I conveyed all my points.

I must admit that it was cathartic to be able to formally share my viewpoints. I was having my own flashbacks to March 2009 when I was on Capitol Hill to speak to congressional offices about pancreatic cancer. In some ways, talking about the mental health needs of the military was harder. Both touched my life very closely and I felt a need and a responsibility to make a difference and help others not just my own family. But talking about PTSD and its impact on military families and lives was a more delicate topic for me for obvious reasons: my concern for confidentiality and privacy.

Perhaps because I think that there is an understanding that military family members are not to speak out, especially to tell Congress that "it is neither ethically nor morally acceptable to send loved ones off to war without the resources that they need to protect themselves,"

I can only guess that others might feel that they cannot talk about the painful changes they are seeing in their loved ones as well. It is a taboo topic filled with stigma, as if our loved ones are weak and not made of the "right stuff" for the military. I wonder if this silence is like a cancer that eats away at our loved ones and our families.

After the briefing, I stayed in the room for an extra 45 minutes taking questions from the audience, including some Senate staffers who were officers in the military. Their stories were so poignant and courageous. I felt like we were their voices and I hope that we did them justice.

The three points that I wanted to make in that briefing room were the following: 1) War changes everyone and people adapt. Those changes are a normal reaction to an abnormal situation with PTSD at the other end of the continuum, where the adaptation process has progressed to a dysfunctional state; 2) We should offer mandatory surveillance and rehabilitation before, during and post-deployment; and 3) Family members need to be involved. Currently we have nowhere to go to confidentially report changes that we see in our loved ones without causing potential damage to their careers.

After the briefing I left the hearing room with Colonel Ireland. We walked together to the train station. I felt a sense of sadness and exhaustion as I entered the Metro. It was an honor to have had the opportunity to speak and share ideas, but the weight of what we still needed to accomplish is monumental.

SHOCK AND AWE

"Shock and awe" is a phrase that was introduced and quickly woven into our conversations during March 2003. We knew that it conveyed our military's strength and superiority fighting the enemy in Iraq. We were transfixed by the fireworks illuminating the night's sky over Baghdad. Years have gone by since "shock and awe" transformed our lexicon and over a decade since our troops landed in Afghanistan. Battles have been fought in distant lands to protect our freedom and security.

Now we are finally acknowledging that this war is coming home. On March 18, 2009, in two locations in our nation's capital, the truth about this war reached our shores. For years we knew that this was coming, but it was difficult to face. The casualties are not just our troops; the collateral damage also includes their families. At the Pentagon, the Secretary of Veterans Affairs and the Deputy Secretary of Defense hosted a screening of the PBS special "Coming Home: Military Families Cope with Change"—a show that highlights families who have faced amputations, traumatic brain injuries and post-traumatic stress disorder. While at the same time, there was a hearing of the Senate Armed Services Committee to discuss the rise of suicides among military personnel.

What connects these two events is shock and AWE. It is time for our nation to accept and understand a new version of this concept—one still grounded in military strength but now associated with a benevolent action rather than destruction. Military jargon is filled with acronyms. So to continue that long-standing tradition, AWE can be an acronym for "Adaptation to the War Environment." AWE is a normal process that the body and psyche experiences to adapt to the extreme environment of battle in order for a person to survive. By just changing the nomenclature, we can begin to change a climate filled with stigma, fear and humiliation. Instead of saying post-traumatic stress disorder or PTSD to describe the signs and symptoms that our troops experience—which can imply victimization, weakness, disability or disease—we can describe it as AWE, a normal reaction to an abnormal situation.

During the Senate hearing, every military leader expressed concern over the soaring rates of military suicides. These rates are higher than the general population despite suicide prevention programs. General Peter W. Chiarelli, Vice Chief of Staff of the Army cited long deployments and separations from family and the perceived stigma and shame associated with getting help. This point was also expressed by Admiral Patrick Walsh, Vice Chief of Naval Operations.

In 2009, General Carter Ham and Brigadier General Gary Patton courageously went public about their reactions to the stress of war and the need for mental healthcare. They wanted to encourage service members to come forward and ask for help. Some junior officers and enlisted personnel may still be reluctant to do this, believing that the generals were able to be open about their situations because they were at the pinnacles of their careers, and if they seek help, they will be passed over for promotions. This perception will be hard to change if the climate is not dramatically altered.

We need to not only provide the superficial modification of wording from PTSD to AWE, but also dispel the notion that only a few are affected by war. Everyone comes back changed. We are fighting an unconventional war. It is now time to take an unconventional approach to prevention and treatment of this issue. Otherwise, we will continue to be a nation haunted by ghosts. I believe that even when our loved ones return, some with physical injuries, it is the invisible injuries that damage the fabric of lives. They may have come home, but emotionally they have disappeared. Family members, holding on to these precious spirits, desperately search for healthcare which could bring back their loved ones. We have created this environment because our mental healthcare programs have failed.

It is time that we come forward and state that we expect that all our troops will return with reactions to the extreme environment of war. It is the norm rather than an abnormality. It then becomes a shared experience and not associated with shame or dishonor. This approach has worked in other settings such as within NASA. For example, it is expected that all astronauts will experience bone loss secondary to the microgravity environment in space. Astronauts undergo training to achieve maximum fitness before they fly, utilize countermeasures such as physical activity during flight to mitigate loss and all go through extensive rehabilitation programs when they return. The severity of the bone loss and recovery varies by astronaut, but they know that they will all lose and will require assistance to protect their health at home and "flight readiness" for their missions.

This model could work for our military. We can help our troops better prepare in advance for the stresses of war, have countermeasures in the field such as well trained mental health personnel and mandatory rehabilitation and surveillance upon return to a non-hostile environment. If we assume that everyone will have adapted to the war environment (AWE) and will require mental healthcare, it removes the stigma associated with it.

This novel approach can help to protect the "fight readiness" of our troops for the battlefield and for their adjustment to the home front. Imagine the day when it will be a badge of courage and honor to say "I'm in AWE."

THE FEMALE WARRIOR

War impacts everyone in the military family—from the warrior to the spouse to the children. For too long the impact of war especially on women, either as the female Service member or the spouse, was negated or ignored. Finally, the Department of Defense, the Veterans Administration and Congress are acknowledging that these wounds need to be evaluated, treated and eventually prevented

The wars in Iraq and Afghanistan were the first that saw a significant number of female troops in combat. As such, they and the military have to deal with seeing war from an entirely new perspective. At the same time, the American public must face the reality of more women being injured and killed in war.

For many years, researchers have looked into how women with TBI fare compared to men with the same condition. Female veterans experiencing TBI have complained about the loss of personal and professional identity, the disruption of family structure, and more common problems from TBI such as fatigue, depression, isolation and changes to self-esteem and sexuality.

Another sad fact of war that female soldiers are facing is amputation. In 2006, the *Washington Post* published an article about amputation and female veterans. The reporter, Donna St. George, profiled a female veteran, Dawn Halfaker. She was severely injured while serving in Iraq, but had warned medics not to cut her arm off. In the end, it was amputated to save her life.

Clearly, amputees have been a part of warfare for as long as it has been recorded in history. When it comes to modern warfare, at least in the United States, female amputees are new. In the Iraq and Afghanistan wars, women were seeing combat unlike any in recent history. Dawn Halfaker was a lieutenant and a patrol leader. The thought of a woman leading a patrol in Vietnam would have been unrealistic.

Lieutenant Halfaker's story touched on how it could be more difficult for women. It is believed that female troops experience more traumas from amputation than their male counterparts because they care more about appearance. I think that statement does a disservice to both men and women. Men may not express it as openly, but I doubt they care less if they lose an arm or a leg. Functional impairment is significant so that even simple activities such as combing one's hair, making a meal, carrying a child, cleaning a gun or tying one's boots are now difficult to perform.

A report from the October 2009 meeting of the Department of Veterans Affairs Advisory Committee on Women Veterans included information on the Prosthetics Women's Workgroup, recognizing the growing number of female veterans. The working group was charged with enhancing the care of female veterans needing a prosthetic. Some of the group's goals are to identify new technologies for women, propose ideas for research, and to support a change in the perception of female veterans through education. From NASA studies on space suits, we know that men and women move body parts differently and that size is not the only issue regarding appropriate fit. These considerations are important to finding the best prosthetic limbs for both men and women.

Amputation is not the only risk faced by the new female soldier. Sadly, one of the most shocking threats to female soldiers in Iraq was from their fellow soldiers. According to a *New York Times* article in May of 2008, "nearly a third of female veterans said they were sexually assaulted or raped while in the military, and 71 percent to 90 percent say they were sexually harassed by the men with whom they served."

A 2009 report by the VA stated that the majority of women serving in the military have faced sexual trauma. Thirty-two percent experienced physical harassment of a sexual nature, 42 percent experienced sexual harassment, and 24 percent experienced rape. These are truly staggering and heartbreaking figures. When someone is serving along side their fellow comrades—putting their life on the line, they need to know that their back is protected and they have support. They should not have fear that their well-being is in jeopardy. The enemy should not be in one's camp or barracks.

What are we doing to stop it? The U.S. Army started the I. A.M. STRONG campaign to fight sexual assaults in the military before they occur. Its core concepts are—Intervene, Act and Motivate. In 2009, Senator Al Franken got an amendment passed that prevents the Defense Department from using contractors to handle sexual assault claims through mandatory employment arbitration. The amendment sprung from the case of Jamie Leigh Jones, who claims to have been raped by other employees while working for Halliburton in Iraq. She was supposedly told she could not file charges and had to pursue her claims through the companies binding arbitration clause.

In December 2009, the military released the Report of the Defense Task Force on Sexual Assault in the Military Services. The task force was created in 2005 and the report examines the progress the military has made since that time. The findings include putting the Sexual Assault Prevention and Response Office directly under the Deputy Secretary of Defense for at least one year. They also found funding for prevention and response programs to be sporadic. One of their more significant findings was that the office did not provide support for victims and, instead, limited itself to handling policy issues. The report suggested establishing a victim advocate position.

The report looked into prevention and training and found that much of the military's efforts at sexual harassment prevention have centered on "bystander intervention." The Task Force went on to recommend that any prevention efforts should "encompass strategic direction, prevention, response, and accountability." The Task Force also had concerns with statistics given during an annual report to Congress and felt the Department of Defense must make real changes to their accountability.

The report concluded that the Department of Defense efforts to address sexual assault in the military is evident since 2005, but also uneven. The Task Force lauded the military's improvements to responding to victims. It ends with a very true statement:

"Our recommendations highlight the need for institutional change to more effectively prevent sexual assault and address related issues. Doing so is not only ethically and morally correct, but also essential to military readiness—all the more critical at this time in our Nation's history."

This is a very real problem facing the military. One study explored the link between sexual trauma and substance abuse. The results of their preliminary study "suggested a high incidence of post-traumatic stress disorder or PTSD related to sexual trauma in a substance-abusing population of female veterans and a high incidence of substance abuse among female veterans who presented requesting help for sexual trauma." A more recent study compared rates of PTSD among female veterans who reported sexual trauma. Almost 200 women completed questionnaires on health and military history. Ninety-two percent reported some kind of trauma and 41 percent reported military sexual trauma specifically. Those reporting sexual trauma had higher rates of PTSD—43 percent to 60 percent. It is clear that women serving in the military are experiencing trauma. Their lives, and the lives of their families, are being affected.

There is no doubt that women in combat situations face an institution that prides itself on tradition and obedience. In a Department of Defense press release dated December 22, 2009, on the prohibition against pregnancy, this was never made clearer. Major Gen. Anthony A. Cucolo III was quoted as saying:

"Anyone who leaves this fight early because they made a personal choice that changed their medical status or contributed to making someone no longer deployable is not in keeping with a key element of the Army's warrior ethos—I will always place the mission first—I believe there should be professional consequences for making a choice like that."

Furthermore, this release stated that Cucolo "formally prohibits soldiers under his command from becoming pregnant or impregnating a soldier." Men, therefore, were at risk of being court-martialed. The risk, however, is not equal considering a woman cannot, in most cases, hide that she is pregnant, but it is more difficult to prove the father. On December 24, 2009, General Ray Odierno stated that the policy, in effect since November 4, 2009, would be lifted as of January 1, 2010 after a public outcry on the absurdity of the situation. This was not a way to improve morale and unit cohesion. Perhaps, providing better education on birth control and safe sexual practices could do more.

The military is facing a whole new set of variables to which it must adjust its policies and programs. For example, they are revising body armor designs to better fit female soldiers. English studies have found that female soldiers are more likely to sustain an injury from military training, work or even recreation. The list could seem endless, but it is heartening to see the Department of Defense take these issues seriously. It cannot be easy for this institution to change. Yet, stressful times can lead to some of the most profound changes. As seen in nature, one needs to adapt to survive and to eventually evolve. The military can do that as well.

HOME FRONT

Women who return from active duty face many additional challenges. The VA reports that the number of homeless female veterans has doubled over the last decade. The GAO estimated that in 2005, 194,000 veterans were homeless on any given night. In fact, now one out of ten homeless veterans under the age of 45 are women. Many of those women have small children.

A VA report from October 2009 states that five percent of homeless veterans are women. It listed risk factors for homelessness as "combat, sexual trauma, poverty, lack of affordable housing, and limited child care support." Clearly two of those factors are specific towards female veterans. The report offers a lower homeless number, 31,000 to the GAO's 194,000. The discrepancy is not unusual. Among affordable housing statistics, homelessness is the hardest to calculate accurately for it can change drastically from night to night, and is difficult to verify.

Women are posing a whole new challenge to the VA. More than ever, they must address issues such as the challenges of being single mothers. Another issue revolves around delivering sex and gender-specific healthcare. VA healthcare has been tailored toward men since its inception. Now, with women comprising over eight percent of veterans, new considerations have to be made.

According to the GAO, over 281,000 women received healthcare from the VA. This number represented a 12 percent increase since 2006. The GAO visited nine VA medical centers (VAMC) and ten community-based outpatient clinics (CBOC) to determine if they were implementing VA policies pertaining to the treatment of women. An example given in the report was that many of the visited facilities did not have "adequate visual and auditory privacy in their check-in areas." For their part, the facilities brought up a valid point. They claimed that space constraints in existing facilities made it difficult to implement many of the privacy policies.

They found that none of the sites had fully implemented the policies. They did find that most were providing basic gender and sex-specific services such as pelvic examinations and access to female healthcare providers. When it came to more complicated issues, such as dealing with abnormal cervical cancer screenings, all the facilities referred patients to non-VA providers.

While big issues face the VA in adjusting to the changing face of the military, some things seem way too simple to overlook. The GAO report from 2009 found that seven of the VAMCs and all ten of the CBOCs did not have sanitary products available in the restrooms. Sometimes, the smallest changes can really make a big difference when it comes to a woman feeling comfortable.

What is disappointing is that the VA had set the bar high to deliver quality healthcare to women in the 1990s. When I was with the Office on Women's Health, we decided to develop National Centers of Excellence in Women's Health based on the model that the VA had established in which 8 VA centers across the nation were deemed worthy to have the VA Center of Excellence in Women's Health designation. Each of these centers provided comprehensive multi-disciplinary care in one setting.

Eventually the VA discontinued these centers, as did the Office on Women's Health. One reason that I was given when I asked why during a congressional hearing was that the VA wanted all its centers to be delivering the quality of care that is associated with a center of excellence. Yet, many female veterans have stated that they want special centers to go to and feel comfortable in. The VA is wrestling with these issues as the female veterans population is increasing.

Female soldiers are not the only ones suffering. Military wives are also showing the effects of war. A study published in the *New England Journal of Medicine* looked at the outpatient medical care data of over 250,000 wives who received care between 2003 and 2006. They found that the deployment of spouses and the length of deployment were associated with depressive disorders, sleep disorders, anxiety, acute stress reactions and adjustment disorders. The diagnosis under every category went up when deployment was greater than 11 months. This study did not include spouses whose husbands were in the National Guard and Reserves. So the numbers may be even higher especially since these groups are not often connected to a military base or a support system.

There is no doubt that spouses and family members of soldiers live under considerable stress. They wait for news of their loved ones, fearing every day they have been injured. Men or women with children with a spouse serving in the military also fear that they will be left to raise their children alone. They often feel alone, convinced that their neighbors and community cannot understand what they are going through. In short, they live under chronic stress, and studies have shown how that can be bad for health.

In 2006, researchers looked at how chronic stress at work affects a subject's health. They measured stress at work for each subject over a 14-year period and found a correlation between work stressors and the risk of metabolic syndrome, a group of disorders such as high blood pressure and cholesterol that promote the development of coronary artery disease. Employees with chronic stress were more than twice as likely to have the syndrome. If such a high increase in risk was reported for work stress, imagine what it might be for families living with the stress of having a loved one face potential physical or psychological harm or even death every day thousands of miles away from home.

Some of the research on military families is heartbreaking. One study looked at the children in military families of enlisted soldiers who saw combat between 2001 and 2004. They explored the correlation between deployment and child maltreatment in 1,771 families. Reports of maltreatment were greater when the solider was deployed to a combat situation.

Another study looked at adolescents of military families. They found that the children exhibited uncertainty about what deployment meant and how it would affect their lives. They did not know what was going to happen to them or their families, and exhibited behavioral changes such as acting out and emotional outbursts. Also, depression and anxiety were common.

An earlier study, however, had a more hopeful finding. Researchers looked at adolescents of military families and the rate of psychopathology. They found that their results did not support the theory that such adolescents are more prone to psychopathology. Among children who had a standardized psychopathology rating scale administered, levels were consistent with studies using nonmilitary groups; and parents' and children's symptom checklist ratings were at national norms. Unfortunately, as the war continues, the negative impact on children's lives will escalate-potentially creating a new lost generation.

Along with having to worry about a spouse in combat overseas, now we have seen that the very home base of many families serving in the military can be unsafe. I was in Berlin when I heard the news about the Fort Hood shootings in 2009. I had been awake for about 40 hours, catching only two hours of sleep the night before while on a plane. I was in Berlin to give a speech at a medical conference. When I arrived at the hotel, I was planning on getting some much needed rest. That was not to be. At 9:30 Berlin time, life changed for all of us with any military connection.

I was getting ready for bed when I had turned on the only English speaking channel. My heart froze as I saw the special news bulletin. Soldiers had been killed and many injured at Fort Hood, Texas. As news unfolded, I could not believe what I was watching. When I learned the perpetrator was a doctor, I was angry. Here was a person that the troops trusted with their lives, and he betrayed them. My heart went out to the families of those soldiers who were killed. These soldiers were home. They were supposed to be safe.

I ended up staying awake all night, transfixed by every news story. In the morning, I headed to my medical conference in a slight daze. I was running on adrenalin and dismay. I kept thinking back to the fact that I had been on the road when a soldier killed his fellow troops overseas in May of 2009. I was on the road once again, and I had an urge to be home, safe, and with the people who would understand how I felt.

The doctor at Fort Hood exhibited some signs of trouble prior to the attack. Such clues cannot be ignored because we need people to fight wars overseas. The war has come home to our shores. I have urged our congressional leaders to make sure that families are included in the assessments of our troops just as their commanders or supervisors need to be more engaged. Families know when things are wrong even when our service members are still able to do their jobs. Families can help protect their loved ones so that they can protect all of us.

There is no doubt that families with loved ones in the military face many hardships. Fortunately, there is now some assistance from the private sector. Organizations such as the Blue Star Families exist to provide support for these families. Blue Star Families was formed in 2008 by military spouses to raise awareness of the challenges faced by military families. They connect fellow military families and the larger community. At the same time, they focus on the positive goals of bringing enjoyment and helpful services to bases. The group has worked with the First Lady, Michelle Obama, on military family issues and presented survey results to several members of Congress on lifestyle concerns.

As the war continues, I continue to hope that our political leaders will translate their verbal commitments into action. The health issues that our veterans face will last for generations to come. I was delighted to hear the First Lady express her support in public and on a heartfelt phone call to military families on Veteran's Day in 2008. I was on that phone call and it meant so much to all of us to know that we had an advocate at the highest level. Dr. Jill Biden, the wife of the Vice President, has also been involved. Her son served in Iraq. It helps that the political power base is aware and active.

Both the White House and the Congress want to appear supportive of military families which can help set the tone for how the rest of the American public responds to the needs of this important group which has often been neglected except for certain holidays such as Veteran's or Memorial Day. Honoring and helping out military families should be a daily commitment by the American public for the sacrifice that these families make.

I have often thought that if there was a draft, hundreds of thousands of Americans or maybe even millions would march in the streets to demand that our troops and their families receive the resources they need to stay healthy and strong. When a war is carried on the backs of less than 1% of the population, it is difficult to get voices raised to be heard. Unfortunately, it often takes tragic events like Fort Hood to set off the alarm that more needs to be done to protect those who protect us.

* * *

For so many with loved ones in the military, the years since September 11, 2001 have been a series of time together, trying to recapture the promise of marriages, the joys of caring for children, the bliss of simple gifts such as taking a walk and vast time apart when are fears are magnified by news reports of bombings and death. The public can understand that finality, but there is another side to this war that is finally being exposed—the psychological and traumatic impairment which can be hard to measure and visualize. It has been stated that cognitive brain injury and post-traumatic stress disorder are the signature injuries of these conflicts.

Even when our loved ones return, some with physical injuries as well, it is these invisible wounds that damage the fabric of lives. They may come home, but emotionally they have disappeared. Military families across this country can share tales of how loved ones cannot sit in crowded rooms or outdoors for fear of an explosive device being detonated. How the nights are filled with terror as images shatter dreams. Perhaps, these are normal reactions to abnormal situations. Yet, these reactions create chaos in the world back home which is not bombarded with enemy fire or bombs.

On September 5, 2008, the Army stated that the suicide rate among returning veterans was higher than the general population and even among Vietnam warriors and these casualties continue to climb—shocking numbers which should have alarmed the American public and created a public outcry. But there were no outcries, not even a whimper.

The years of planning and leading missions, evading or stalking an enemy, always being on guard have taken a massive toll on our loved ones' psyches and their health as well as their families. Then to navigate healthcare systems that don't acknowledge these injuries for concern over disability payments or ineptitude only compound a tragic situation. I recall speaking to one Vet Center health provider who told me that their goal was to keep our troops off the streets and out of jail-lofty goals for our citizens who have defended our nation.

We must stop viewing the treatment of invisible injuries as a luxury. It is a necessity to ensure that our troops, our loved ones, can defend our nation and come back and be productive members of our society and our families. It has taken a nation of ghosts—individuals coming back from wars with their spirits and bodies broken to finally achieve this call to arms.

Stellar Questions:

How can someone help a military family in the neighborhood?

If you know a family that has a loved one serving in the military, consider asking if there's anything you can do to help or invite them to join your family for a meal, or just a cup of coffee. As a country at war— with so many reservists and National Guard involved—there isn't always the traditional military community out there to support families. Isolation, loneliness and fear are emotions that are hard to share with those who are not experiencing the same situations. By offering a warm hug, a cup of coffee, or a meal to share is a great gift that can mean so much.

At the same time, be informed. Talk to your elected officials about veterans' healthcare and reach out to a local advocacy group that supports military families to see if you can help. There are many groups that have formed over the years and they provide a diverse array of services. At the very least, keep informed. Know what is going on and share your opinion on the issues. The worst thing we can do for our troops is to ignore their struggles by being silent.

What is a Center of Excellence in Traumatic Brain Injury and why do we need them?

The Department of Defense (DOD) released a press release on November 30, 2007, announcing the creation of a Center of Excellence to address traumatic brain injury (TBI). It represented "a national collaborative network to advance and disseminate TBI knowledge, enhance clinical and management approaches, and facilitate other vital services to best serve the urgent and enduring needs of warrior families with TBI."

The Center of Excellence is a joint effort between DOD and the VA. It is an effort to focus a large amount of research into psychological health and TBI. Through qualified practitioners, they will look at prevention of injury and resilience to combat stress. One objective is to cut the time it takes a soldier to get through the system, from injury to receiving benefits, in half. One positive aspect of the effort is the cooperation between the two agencies.

There is no doubt that such a center is necessary. The new state of warfare has increased the likelihood of TBI. Between the prevalence of explosive injuries and the fact that body armor is helping soldiers survive injuries that in the past would have been fatal, the development of the center is a logical improvement to healthcare for veterans, and another example of the military adapting to the new face of war.

What is a Vet Center and is it the same as a VA clinic?

The VA established a series of community centers called Vet Centers. They provide confidential counseling and employment assistance to service members who served in combat and to their families. Centers are staffed by small teams, many of them veterans. There are 232 Vet Centers in the nation.

The VA offers community based outpatient clinics. There are 800 sites that provide common outpatient services, including wellness visits. The big difference between VA clinics and Vet Centers is in the type of services and the degree of patient confidentiality they provide. Clinics focus on health issues while centers focus more on helping those returning from combat readjust to civilian living conditions.

Should women be on the front lines in combat?

A 1994 Pentagon policy restricts female soldiers from being on the front line. The concept of a front line drastically changed during the wars in Afghanistan and Iraq. The idea that the U.S. military will face another enemy across a defined boundary may never happen again.

I believe that women should serve right beside men. I think about Major Jennifer Snyder. She was the first women to be awarded the Silver Star for her involvement in a battle near Baghdad. She was also cited for heroism in close combat. Female troops have risked their lives in these wars and should be acknowledged for their skills and bravery.

Should women be allowed to defer deployment if they have young children?

It is reported that over 100,000 mothers have served in these recent wars which is nearly half the total number of women deployed. These mothers are torn between serving and being with their children. The Army, for their part, needs to keep enlistment up, and has changed some of its policies to ease the stress on mothers.

In 2008, the time a new mother can defer deployment was increased from four to six months. There may be some flexibility in this policy as a base commander of a medical center in Germany has extended that time to a year. The Army approved a 10-day paternity leave for new fathers as well.

There is no doubt that mothers with young children face a difficult transition when deployed. At the same time, when a service member enlists, they do so knowing that when you are deployed, you need to obey your orders.

How do I know if my spouse has PTSD/AWE or TBI?

According to the Mayo Clinic, the symptoms of PTSD can include the following:

Flashbacks or reliving traumatic events for up to days at a time.
Upsetting dreams about traumatic event.
Avoidance of thinking about or talking about the event.
Feeling emotionally numb.
Avoiding activities once enjoyed.
Hopelessness.
Memory troubles.
Relationship troubles.
Irritability.
Overwhelming guilt or shame.
Self-destructive behavior—drinking too much alcohol.
Trouble sleeping.
Easy to startle or frighten.
Hearing or seeing things that are not there.

According to the Mayo Clinic, the symptoms of TBI can include:
Mild TBI

>Brief unconsciousness.
>Amnesia of events.
>Right before and after the event.
>Dizziness or loss of balance.
>Blurred vision, ringing in ears or bad taste to mouth.
>Mood changes.
>Memory or concentration problems.

Moderate to Severe TBI

>Persistent headache.
>Repeated vomiting or nausea.
>Convulsions or seizures.
>Inability to awaken from sleep.
>Dilation of one or both pupils of the eyes.
>Slurred speech.
>Weakness or numbness in the extremities.
>Loss of coordination.
>Profound confusion.
>Agitation, combativeness.

Try to find a provider who specializes in PTSD or TBI. The two conditions can be tied together, and both can be difficult to diagnose. There are some new experimental tests that measure brain function to assess whether a person has PTSD. Additionally, new functional brain imaging may help to diagnose TBI. These tests may help us to improve the diagnosis and treatment of patients who suffer from these conditions.

The long-term impact of TBI can include neurocognitive changes such as memory impairment, vestibular or balance disorders, hearing deficits, adjustment disorders and PTSD. Even though mild TBI which is a different entity from severe TBI can resolve, some cases just like PTSD may present months or even years after the traumatic event. Additionally, toxins in the environment can cause TBI especially in patients who have been exposed to prior head trauma and are more susceptible.

What is the association between space travel and mild TBI?

Astronauts when they launch into space and then return to Earth face significant G forces or forces of gravity on their bodies. The brain in these situations can experience an acceleration/de-acceleration type injury resulting in mild TBI. Astronauts may complain of dizziness and trouble walking when they return from space flight with symptoms more severe after long flights. There may be additional injury to the brain from radiation exposure which is greater in space than on Earth or from toxins found in the space vehicle. Astronauts are checked for neuro-vestibular changes such as dizziness immediately upon return to Earth and undergo rehabilitation if there are any deficits detected. The brain injuries seen in the astronauts may be similar to what is seen in troops returning from battle. The military and space communities may be valuable partners in helping the civilian population better diagnose and treat TBI.

Should there be a draft and, if so, should women be included?

If a war is essential for our country to fight, I believe there should be a draft. If there is a draft, women should be included. I believe in equality in the workforce and that extends to our military as well.

I respect Israel's policy on military service. It is mandatory for both men and women after they graduate from high school. Men serve for 36 months and women for 21 months. Both can be excused for medical or religious reasons. Married women can be excused which I don't think is necessary. After serving, men are required to provide 45 days a year for reserve duty until they are 40. Some women are required to serve in the reserves as well, until they are 26 years old. With such a policy, I believe it would ensure that every war we decide to enter would be worth the fight. A draft could further unite the nation with this shared experience.

Do we need private programs such as "To Give an Hour" to help our troops?

To Give an Hour is a not-for-profit organization that was developed by Dr. Barbara Van Dahlen to "develop national networks of volunteers capable of responding to both acute and chronic conditions that arise in our society." This group is focused on helping troops and their families get the mental health services they need. They provide counseling, and treatment for anxiety, depression, substance abuse, PTSD, TBI, sexual health and intimacy concerns, and loss and grieving. It was established to help fill in the gaps that exist in the care of our military members. It is unreasonable to think that the government can do it alone. There are just too many people who need care. There are other programs that have developed in the private sector to help our troops and their families. I believe that public-private programs are important. The needs of our troops and vets cannot be managed by just the government. We all need to help and participate.

Why do military wives feel like that they can't share their concerns about their spouses?

It has often been the tradition that military spouses which usually had been wives were to stay silent and buck it up when they faced adversity. The wife was the representative of the service member. In the military culture, even the rank of the service member conveyed status to the wife—such that an officer's or commander's wife was given a great deal of respect and she had responsibilities to ensure that the unit's families were taken care of during deployments. Until the wars in Iraq and Afghanistan, discourse on TBI or PTSD was not spoken about in public circles—it was often associated with stigma and weakness. Now that even generals have shared their experiences, there is an environment of more openness. However, it needs the test of time to prove that there will be no negative repercussions on careers and promotion.

The military has created Military OneSource which provided services and referrals to military members and their families. Yet, some of the hotlines have disclaimers that what is discussed may be shared with supervisors or commanders. This conveys a feeling that "what you say can and will be use against you." Not a very supportive approach especially if one's commander is not enlightened to the issues. Chaplains have also been more involved with family members' concerns and this may help to dissipate some of the feelings of isolation and fear, especially if chaplains can be an interface between the family and command.

What programs are available to help children with military parents?

According to a Pentagon survey, six out of ten military parents report that their children are experiencing more fear and anxiety when a parent is deployed. One in four parents are concerned that their children have not coped well with the deployment.

The National Child Traumatic Stress Network was established by Congress in 2000. It is a network of academic and community-based service centers. They provide support services to military children and families. The Center for the Study of Traumatic Stress and Families Overcoming Under Stress (FOCUS) also provides assistance to military families.

Operation Military Kid was started by the Army to support children impacted by deployment. Since 2005, they have helped 88,000 children. They offer a variety of recreational and educational programs, and "hero packs" which include fun activities and ways to stay connected with a deployed parent. Every branch has programs to support families. In fact, the Air Force launched in 2010 "The Year of the Family" to highlight programs that provide housing, education, healthcare and childcare. It is also important for schools and community and religious groups to understand the needs of children whose parents are deployed.

CHAPTER SEVEN
SEX, CHOCOLATE, WINE, AND SHOPPING
—Health Benefits of Life's Pleasures

"And in the sweetness of friendship let there be laughter and the sharing of pleasures. For in the dew of little things the heart finds its morning and is refreshed."

—Kahlil Gibran, *The Prophet*

In 2 January 2006, my mother was wrongly put in a hospice. She was placed there following a fall that broke her right hip and arm. Because of her underlying lung condition—she had asthma, bronchitis and scar tissue from a prior lung infection, her primary care doctor did not think that she would survive surgery and that it was more humane to put her in a hospice where she would receive morphine. I was out of the country when she was placed there. I remember that at the time, I reacted as a daughter, not as a doctor. As soon as I returned to the United States, I flew immediately to Denver, where I sat at her bedside for hours feeling helpless. I kept telling myself that there was no way my mother was going to die from a broken hip and arm, but it didn't look good.

After five days, I still had not left her side. When I finally forced myself outside, I found it was freezing. Snow started to fall. I had rushed home from a trip to the Caribbean and was woefully unprepared for the weather. The cold seemed to cut through the adrenaline I had been living on, and I realized I hadn't eaten in some time. My husband and father were there with me and they looked no better. I knew it was time for a change in scenery. I looked up at them and suggested a shopping trip. I needed something warm, especially if the snow was going to continue. We all needed a break.

That day, we spent an hour at a nearby mall. The place was actually closing but a Target store still had its doors open, so we went in. We pushed a cart up and down the aisles, looking for warm clothes, boots, anything we thought we needed. As we walked, I was away from death and dying, and could see there was still life in the world. It was immediately cathartic and my pace quickened. By the time I found the shoe department I was already feeling a little better. When I saw the pair of fleece-lined boots seemingly waiting for my arrival, I knew we had made the right decision. I got a little shopper's high when I saw they were in my size and on sale.

As the three of us continued around the store together, our thoughts cleared and we became united in our plans for what we wanted to do next for my mother. By the time we got back in the car, we were energized and ready to face the hospice. We planned to kidnap my mother and get her back to the hospital where she could get the care she needed to live.

* * *

Not all our troubles are as serious as the illness of a loved one, but for many, fears of greater or lesser degree nag us every day. When our thoughts circle the same path with no relief, it is time to stop and allow ourselves a moment's pleasure. Experiencing pleasure, if only for an hour, breaks the tension in our bodies and allows us to think in new ways. One truly pleasurable way to take a break is to shop, but there are a few others I like to suggest to people. Although at first blush, these may seem like vices, they actually have been found to provide some health benefit. Let's look at some of my favorites:

SEX

I remember watching a very compelling story on the National Geographic channel. The show focused on monkeys, particularly the Bonobo. It is a relative of the chimpanzee. Unlike the chimp, researchers have claimed that the Bonobos are peaceful creatures. In fact, observers claim that to resolve conflict, the Bonobos often use sexual contact. Although some scientists are questioning this aspect of their nature, I still love the idea. Make love, not war.

Once I did a talk about sex and heart health in Idaho. Of course, I was referring to the differences and similarities between men and women as it pertained to cardiovascular disease. A reporter in the audience, however, took some liberties. I picked up the local paper the next day and the byline was: "Doc Says Sex Is Good For A Woman's Heart." This was when I was working for a conservative administration. I was a little worried.

From medical school on, I learned how important sex is to patients, but it was not a topic that we were comfortable discussing. I remember when I was at the University of California, San Francisco. We were doing rounds with one of the top cardiologists in the country. He could put his hand on a patient's chest and tell his or her ejection fraction which tells how well the heart is pumping out blood to the rest of the body. While we were walking the hospital corridor he asked us, "After a heart attack, can a patient have sex?" At first we were surprised. We thought he'd ask a much more technically challenging and important question. He told us just how important a question that is— to the patient. It really hit home for me.

There is no doubt that simply saying the word "sex" draws interest, positive or negative, from most listeners. That's why certain advertisers jump at the chance to use sex to sell products, and why people prove them right by buying those products. At the same time, getting a politician to say the word is pretty difficult unless they have to admit to their own sexual indiscretions.

What I find even more interesting than the politics is the potential health benefits of sex. Many researchers have investigated this and come up with some compelling results. According to two researchers, David G. Blanchflower and Andrew J. Oswald, sex may generate more happiness than money. Although they caution that the statistical results of their work should be treated with caution, they found that sex factored strongly into people's sense of happiness. Ironically, they also found that money did not buy more sex.

Who knows if people really want sex more than money, but that's not the only finding. Sex has also been found to be a painkiller as well. One study showed that genital stimulation by women masked the feeling of pain. The pleasure derived could elevate pain thresholds, but it also activated an analgesic process that was distinct from simple distraction. Another researcher, however, compared the benefits of intercourse as related to masturbation. Researchers compared the amount of prolactin released following intercourse as compared to masturbation and found the levels of the prior 400 percent greater. Prolactin is a hormone in the brain associated with a sense of pleasure and human connection. The findings claim that sexual intercourse is more physiologically satisfying.

Even with this research, some think sex can be dangerous. Who hasn't seen a man keel over during the middle of sex with a massive heart attack on TV or in the movies? Recent research has found that sex isn't as dangerous as once thought, either—at least for men. Not only did they find that frequent sexual intercourse does not increase the risk of stroke for middle-aged men, it also provides "some protection from fatal coronary events." Researchers found that mortality risk was 50 percent lower for men who had frequent orgasms. Imagine the lines a man could now use to entice his partner to have sex with him?

To add to our healthy view of sex, it might also be good for our immune system. Scientists looked at 112 college students and categorized them by how frequently they had sexual encounters. Saliva samples were then taken and tested for immunoglobulin A. Those having frequent encounters were found to have significantly higher levels of this antibody that can protect against infections.

Sex can be good for your blood pressure as well. In one study, the researcher asked subjects to keep a diary of their daily sexual activity. After analyzing the data, he found that people who had intercourse showed a reduction in blood pressure.

It's not just sex, either. Intimacy has been shown to have health benefits as well. It has been long understood how important simple touch is to children. One study augmented the regular hospital care for premature babies with massage four times a day. The children that received the massage showed significantly better weight gain.

It is true for women too. Researchers looked at blood pressure and oxytocin levels of 59 premenopausal women before and after physical intimacy (hugging) with their husbands. They found that frequent hugs by a spouse lead to lower blood pressure and higher oxytocin levels for these women.

During labor, oxytocin is released in high levels after the cervix and vagina distend. It has also been found to be one of the hormones released during sex. In fact, one study investigated it as the possible explanation of sex being a pain killer. Scientists took 48 healthy volunteers and pricked their fingers, judging their pain sensitivity. They then had the volunteers inhale oxytocin. When they inhaled enough to produce a sense of smell, researchers found their pain threshold had increased by over 50 percent.

Others refer to oxytocin as the love hormone. Scientists looked into the biological basis of trust among humans. Their work focused on oxytocin, already known to play a role in social attachment among animals. They found that it also caused a "substantial increase in trust among humans."

Oxytocin is not the only chemical thought to play a role in the positive effects of sex on the body. One researcher at the State University of New York has an interesting take on what sex does for a woman's mood. Gordon Gallup, Ph.D. surveyed 293 women and found that women who did not use a condom during sex were less depressed than women who did, or women who abstained. He also found that those women not using condoms became more depressed the longer they went between sexual encounters. The conclusion he drew from his findings might not be what you expect. It wasn't that the pleasure of sex caused the happiness, nor was it any endorphins or oxytocin the woman's body produced. Instead, he believes that it is the semen. Semen contains sex hormones including testosterone and estrogen. He believes these hormones affect a women's mood, thus women using condoms do not experience the same benefit. Although he claims to have controlled for many variables, there is no way to rule out that whatever personality type chooses to not have protected sex could also be a personality type that is less depressed. Either way, it is a compelling thought. But it goes against what I advise people with partners that may not be monogamous which increases the risk of sexually transmitted diseases.

There is little doubt among women when it comes to the importance of touch. I remember when my mother was in intensive care. We had to wear gowns and gloves because she had a hospital acquired infection. It broke my heart because she had already lost all other comforts. There is a basic human need to be held, to feel the warmth of someone's skin against yours and this was taken away from her as we often do with so many patients in medical facilities to decrease the spread of infections.

This need will soon have to be addressed for space travel too. In the future, we may see privately funded hotels in space. People who can pay a hefty sum will launch into space for a few days circling the Earth every 90 minutes. Now that the private sector is involved, these kinds of issues will be addressed perhaps more openly. Thoughts of sex in space fuel the imagination. Talk about a destination wedding or honeymoon or adventure holiday. The sky will no longer be the limit but our entire galaxy.

CHOCOLATE

Before the war in Iraq in 2003, news stories were encouraging people to make a safe room in their houses. They suggested taping plastic over doors and windows. I made the comment to colleagues that maybe there was a better option. Perhaps we should just go out and buy some chocolate and wine. Rent a movie and curl up on the couch with someone we loved. Maybe that would help more than duct tape and plastic. At least we wouldn't die by suffocation. The element of fear which helped to lead the population towards support of a war was an effective device for manipulation, but destructive for health and wellness.

Although I mentioned chocolate in jest, there are health benefits to this most wonderful of food groups. In fact, astronauts also love chocolate. Space travel affects their ability to taste food. It is thought that the increased blood flow to the head impacts the olfactory system, much like what a cold can do to your taste buds. Due to this, they look for food with a lot of flavor. Spicy food and chocolate are favorites.

Shannon Lucid said that she took M&Ms on her mission to the Mir space station. I can guarantee that if I ever get the joy of traveling into space, chocolate will be in my provisions. My colleagues at NASA know this about me. One holiday season, they sent me boxes and boxes of it. A good friend of mine also sent me a plaque that read, "Chocolate is the thinking woman's aphrodisiac." I have to agree.

Chocolate was first made from the beans from the cacao tree about 2,000 years ago. Early inhabitants of Mexico and Central America, including the Mayans and Aztecs, used the seeds of the tree to make a drink. The Spanish brought it to Europe where its use expanded. Now, according to a Packaged Food report, the United State's market for chocolate is estimated to be near $20 billion in 2011.

Women of the world rejoiced back in the early years of the 21st century. Science came forth with some of the best news ever—chocolate can be healthy. Chocolate contains hundreds of compounds such as serotonin serving as a natural anti-depressant, Theobromine acting like a stimulant much like caffeine, and even endorphins providing a sense of well-being. Studies have found that chocolate can be an antioxidant and may reduce blood pressure. They found that among elderly, previously untreated hypertensive patients, a "calorie-balanced increase in consumption" could reduce blood pressure. I like to view chocolate as nature's gift to humanity.

In both studies, only dark chocolate showed potential health benefits, not white or milk chocolate. Why is dark chocolate different? For one thing, it contains a higher percentage of cacao. Flavanol antioxidants are found in cacao but they give dark chocolate its bitter taste. This bitterness has been combated by chocolate manufacturers, often through harsh processing or masking flavors by adding milk and sugar. This process has been found to reduce the antioxidant level in the chocolate. Some studies have even posited that not all dark chocolates are the same.

Understand this does not give the health conscious carte blanche to eat an unlimited amount of chocolate. I had a patient come in one day who was so excited. She had eaten one of those huge chocolate bars and figured she must be one of the healthiest people on the planet afterwards. You have to be careful how much you eat. The health benefits can quickly be overruled by the sugar and fat and calories usually found in chocolate. I suggest one square or truffle a day.

WINE

Recently, wine and space had a meeting. Richard Mathies, a researcher from Berkley, California noticed he got a headache when he drank red wine. Wondering what it was, he asked a colleague who mentioned it may be due to Tyramine, an amino acid that creates adrenaline. When he decided that was a problem, he wanted to figure out which foods contained Tyramine. He was the perfect person to do it.

Dr. Mathies was working on the Mars Organic Analyzer. It could be the most sensitive tool in trying to detect life on the red planet. Using his prototype, he analyzed wine. He found merlots to be particularly high in Tyramine. Someday, a smaller version of the analyzer may be used by people with food sensitivities. It's another example of how NASA research eventually leads to everyday advances in science.

At home, we often had red wine at the dinner table—sometimes watered down with seltzer. My father is from Cluj, Romania. He always told me that wine was good for you. He was right, as long as we don't overdo it.

Even more than the other "delights" that society labels as a vice, wine personifies the importance of moderation. It is generally accepted that drinking too much alcohol causes damage to a number of our internal organs, not least of which the liver. It can increase blood pressure, contribute to obesity and cause accidents. However, researchers have found that drinking red wine in moderation can actually provide health benefits. Researchers have looked at a number of compounds found in red wine as the source of these benefits. One such chemical is resveratrol. It comes from the skin of the grape and is one of the many active, non-alcoholic ingredients in red wine. The reason red wine has more than white wine is that it is fermented with the skin longer. One study isolated it as possibly preventing cancer, as well as protecting heart and brain function. One of the authors of the study, Lindsay Brown, is quoted as saying that resveratrol "turns on the cell's own survival pathways, preventing damage."

Red wine also contains antioxidants. According to the Mayo Clinic, compounds in the wine can increase the levels of good cholesterol such as high-density lipoproteins and protect against artery damage. These compounds come in two varieties, flavonoids and non-flavonoids.

The Mayo Clinic also points out that drinking any kind of alcohol in moderation can help the heart. It has been found to raise the "good" cholesterol, reduce blood clots and help prevent plaque formation in arteries. Alcohol decreases a protein that stimulates smooth muscle cells in coronary arteries that can lead to plaques or blockages. It's important to note that the American Heart Association does not recommend the consumption of alcohol to prevent heart disease.

If you already drink wine, stick to moderation—two drinks a day for men, one for women. According to the CDC, the standard drink in the United States is equal to 0.6 ounces of pure alcohol. This translates to 12 ounces of beer, 8 ounces of malt liquor, 5 ounces of wine, or 1.5 ounces of 80 proof distilled spirits or liquor. The discrepancy between the sexes relates to men being, on average, larger than women and, according to the National Institute on Alcohol Abuse and Alcoholism, men have more water in their body than women, which helps dilute the alcohol. Women may also metabolize alcohol differently through the liver because of the impact of estrogen on liver enzymes. It takes less alcohol for a woman to become inebriated compared to a man.

It is important to point out that scientists are investigating another danger from alcohol consumption. Studies have found a link between even moderate drinking and an increased risk of breast, pancreatic and liver cancer. The Department of Health and Human

Services has even listed alcohol as a known human carcinogen. The Canadian Centre for Addiction and Mental Health found that people who stop drinking can reduce their risk of head and neck cancer. It is suggested that women consume more foods such as leafy green vegetables that contain folate and other B vitamins or B vitamin supplements which impact cell division to offset the potentially carcinogenic effects of alcohol.

SHOPPING

When thinking about hotels in space, I like to take it another step and envision shopping among the stars someday. Can you imagine the souvenirs you would bring back? Since there is less gravity on the moon or on the space station compared to Earth, bags filled with items would not be heavy. There would also be no customs tax upon return to the planet.

Just like the other "vices" discussed in this chapter, shopping has its issues. I remember in 2004, I was giving a talk at an American Heart Association event. Prior to the date, the organizer called my office and asked my secretary, a man, what I like to do. He answered, "Shopping." In retrospect, I think that he said that because of his stereotype of women and he knew that his wife liked to shop.

When I arrived at the venue, I had no idea they had called and talked to my secretary. The director of the association stood up to introduce me. After going through my biography, he ended by saying, "…and she likes to shop."

I was shocked. I had never been introduced like that before. I was surprised that was what my secretary shared with him. To save face, I modified my speech and talked about the health benefits of shopping. The event closed with a silent auction. One of the baskets for sale was filled with chocolates, wine and cheese—everything that I loved. I encouraged the audience to shop—it would not only support the Association but it would improve their health.

One of my favorite places to shop is the hardware store. I know that it sounds odd, but it's really the best equal opportunity environment to shop in. Men and women can enjoy walking down rows and rows filled with equipment, tools, household items, and paints galore. I find it to be an empowering place especially as a woman. It makes me feel like I can take care of myself. I smile when I think that two of the best gifts I have ever been given were a power drill and a lawn mower. I remember being so disappointed when the hardware shop near my house closed its doors.

Even shopping at the mall can be good for you. Walking and carrying bags is a weight bearing exercise which is good for bone health. During wonderful sales, you move faster to get there so there is aerobic exercise which improves heart health and can expend calories to help decrease weight. Also, women tend to shop in groups which increase oxytocin levels and lower cortisol or stress hormone levels. Just like for other physical activity, I like to recommend shopping at least thirty minutes a day for most days of the week and it does not need to be done all at the same time.

Scientific studies support my recommendations. Some researchers have found that shoppers can get a high. It is thought that while shopping, at least for some people, the brain releases dopamine, a chemical in the brain associated with pleasure. Much as it does for addictive behaviors, dopamine makes us feel good and want to do it again.

Another aspect of shopping that could be of some benefit has to do with who shops with you. One researcher, Paco Underhill, has been very active in studying human behavior in a retail environment. In his book, *Why We Shop—the Science of Shopping*, he relates his findings that when two women shop together, they shop much longer than if they are with a man or with children. Interestingly, according to his findings, women shop the shortest amount of time when accompanied by a man, even shorter than when shopping alone. Perhaps that finding could change if it took place in a hardware store.

ADDICTION

The key to almost everything is moderation. I would never recommend getting drunk a couple of times a week, going into debt shopping, eating pounds of chocolate a day or partaking in unsafe or hurtful sexual encounters. If you look at sex, chocolate, wine and shopping, they all have something in common with addictive behavior. That is why moderation is even more important, regardless of the health benefits outlined above.

According to the National Institute on Alcohol Abuse and Alcoholism, alcoholism is defined as a disease with four symptoms: craving, loss of control, physical dependence and tolerance. In short, alcohol significantly reduces the quality of the abuser's life. Right now, there is no cure, but it can be treated with counseling and medications.

The medications address the addiction in different ways. One, Naltrexone, reduces the craving in brain for people who have quit. Another, Acamprosate reduces "detox" symptoms, and Disulfiram can make a person feel sick if they consume alcohol.

With alcohol, even moderation has to be undertaken responsibly. The National Institute on Alcohol Abuse and Alcoholism recommends that people not drink at all if they are pregnant, plan to drive, taking certain over-the-counter medications, recovering alcoholics and/or under the age of 21.

Alcoholism is a disease and it can be inherited. Alcoholics cannot have even one drink. One study investigating alcoholism found an interesting correlation between eating and the disease. They found that ghrelin, a hormone that the stomach produces to increase hunger, may play a part in alcohol reward. In addition, they found that inhibiting that hormone could suppress alcohol consumption. If ghrelin plays a part in rewarding an addictive behavior, it could be an interesting link between alcoholism and overeating.

Speaking of overeating, everyone knows someone that is a chocoholic. The word is used in jest; and chocolate addiction is not an established diagnosis; however, there is some basis for the claim. One study investigated chocolate cravings. They found that the "psychopharmacologic and chemosensory effects of chocolate must be considered when formulating recommendations for overall healthy eating." What they are saying is that the fat and sugar found in chocolate combined with the texture and aroma of the experience of eating chocolate, then added to its apparent mood-altering affects, should be considered similar to the experience addicts get from other sources such as alcohol, drugs and sex.

Dopamine was one of the chemicals researchers investigated when reviewing the data on chocolate cravings. It is a neurotransmitter that is closely tied to addiction. It has been tied to feelings of enjoyment and reinforcement in the brain. Many drugs such as cocaine and nicotine increase dopamine levels in the brain. It is no wonder that if dopamine has been tied to chocolate that an addiction may in fact be a real thing.

Like many other addictive behaviors, shopping can increase dopamine levels as well. Compulsive buying disorder is a condition where shopping habits affect someone's quality of life. According to one review, it has a life-time prevalence of 5.8 percent in the United States. Interestingly, sufferers of this disorder seem to be more susceptible to other Axis I disorders—mood disorders, or obsessive-compulsive disorders (OCD), binge eating and substance abuse disorders. One study looked at the available data and came to the conclusion that compulsive shopping could be considered as "compensatory buying that temporarily alleviates depressive symptoms" and that treatment of the underlying depression might alleviate the symptoms of compulsive buying.

The key to any addiction is the effect it has on the health or quality of life of the sufferers or others that he or she encounters. Sometimes that is harder to define than in others. Sexual addiction falls into that category. Not everyone agrees that sexual addiction exists, or if it is a compulsion, or just impulse behavior. Researchers looking at available data felt that the concept of sexual addiction has "uncertain scientific value." One study, that defines sexual compulsion as "a failure to resist the impulse of sex," looked at whether drugs useful in treating other urge-driven conditions—opioid antagonists—are useful to treat the condition. They gave subjects Naltrexone and found that "symptoms drastically decreased and psychosocial functioning improved" while on the medication. Naltrexone is usually used to manage alcohol dependence; therefore, it could make you think it is not so far removed from the addictive properties associated with alcoholism.

* * *

This is my prescription for good health—a glass of wine on occasion with a daily piece of dark chocolate, 30 minutes a day of responsible shopping to get your body moving, and at least a hug a day. What a wonderful new prescription for good health and one that probably will have excellent compliance. It is hard to argue with these doctor's orders!

Stellar Questions:

How can I make shopping healthy?

Here are some suggestions:

Start far away: Park as far away from the entrance as possible. It will add mileage to your exercise and reduce the stress of jockeying for a closer spot.

Take a few laps before you buy anything: If you keep a good pace as you walk the perimeter of the mall, you can get your heart rate up. Also, it's a great chance to window shop.

Keep track of your steps: While at the mall, find the sports store and buy a pedometer. Set a goal of walking 10,000 steps a day.

Make it weight-bearing: When you fill your bags, distribute the weight evenly between both arms. It makes your trip healthier for your bones, joints and muscles.

When you try on clothes, pretend that you are in your own private studio—listen to the music, dance a little or sway your arms—just move. Your body is designed for that—shopping is a great tool to help you do it! Enjoy and remember—a one dollar item can give you just as much pleasure as a $1,000 item too!

Do condoms protect against sexually transmitted disease?

According to the CDC, latex condoms, if used correctly, are highly effective at preventing HIV and can prevent other sexually transmitted diseases. Lab tests have shown that condoms form an "essentially" impermeable barrier to sexually transmitted disease pathogens. They provide less protection, however, from ulcer diseases such as the Human Papilloma Virus (HPV) that also causes genital warts and the Herpes Simplex Virus (HSV) that causes vesicles. Epidemiologic studies are less useful because they cannot control for subjects proper and consistent use of condoms.

The most reliable way to avoid sexually transmitted diseases is through abstaining from sex which may not be realistic or even good for a person's well-being. The second best is to be in a long-term mutually monogamous relationship with a healthy partner. If your partner has an STD, you need to have frank discussion about your risk of getting infected and how to protect yourself from infection if at all possible.

How often should women get pap smears if they sexually active?

Most cervical cancers start in the lining of the cervix. It generally takes time for these cells to develop from precancerous to cancerous. Additionally, the body can repair some of the precancerous changes due to the HPV, and treatment may not be necessary. So less frequent testing is now recommended to avoid unnecessary procedures and anxiety.

The America College of Obstetrics and Gynecology recommends that all women should get screened for cervical cancer at age 21 and be screened every two years until the age of 30. At 30, women who have three normal test results in a row can be tested every three years. Women with risk factors such as diethylstilbestrol (DES) exposure before birth, a history of cervical cancer and those with weakened immune systems, should continue to be tested more frequently. At 65-70, if a woman has had three or more normal results in a row and no abnormal results in ten years may choose to stop getting tested.

What roles does oxytocin play in the body?

Oxytocin is a hormone best known for its role in lactation. Oxytocin is responsible for the letdown reflex in pregnant women. When it acts on the mammary glands, milk becomes available for breast feeding. The act of feeding causes more of the hormone to be released. It also plays a role in cervical dilation during birth.

It was found in 1906 and has since been studied for its role in reproduction. Now, researchers are also looking at what the hormone does in the brain. It has been implicated in learning, anxiety, feeding and pain perception, but also in social behaviors such as trust. It has been shown to be important to social memory and attachment as well as sexual and maternal behavior. According to a review of data, it has recently been associated with autism and schizophrenia.

Does other alcohol provide the same benefits as wine?

According to the Mayo Clinic, moderate alcohol consumption, whether wine or not, can have health benefits. They can include reducing the risk of heart disease and the risk of dying from a heart attack. It might reduce the risk of strokes. It can lower the risk of gallstones and the risk of developing diabetes. Moderate consumption is defined as two drinks a day for men 65 and younger or one drink a day for women and men 66 and older.

On the flip side, they also provide the health risks of excessive drinking. These include cancer of the pancreas, mouth, neck, head, liver and breast. Also, in people with high levels of triglycerides, it can increase the risk of pancreatitis. Alcohol can contribute to sudden death in people with cardiovascular disease which is know as "holiday heart" because of increased drinking during the holidays. It increases the risk of miscarriage and fetal alcohol syndrome. Cognitively, it can lead to injuries from accidents and impaired driving skills as well as suicide especially since it is a depressant. If a woman is pregnant or has an addiction to alcohol, she should not drink.

Does eating leafy greens lower the breast cancer risk for women who drink alcohol?

A report has shown that more than three glasses of alcohol a week are associated with higher breast cancer rates. According to a study highlighted by the American Cancer Society, not eating enough green leafy vegetables if you consume alcohol could increase the risk of developing breast cancer. Leafy green vegetables contain folate and other B vitamins which could counteract some of the negative effects of alcohol. So perhaps a salad with a glass of wine may not be such a bad combination.

**CHAPTER EIGHT
THE STARDUST CONNECTION
—Spirituality, Faith, and Healing**

"The non-violence practiced by men like Gandhi and King may not have been practical or possible in every circumstance, but the love that they preached—their fundamental faith in human progress—that must always be the North Star that guides us on our journey."

—President Barack Obama
2009 Nobel Peace Prize acceptance speech

When NASA celebrated the 40th anniversary of the moon landing, there were many stories written about the lives of the astronauts who made the journey. There is no doubt that the Apollo astronauts returned as conquering heroes to the accolades of an adoring public. The space race captivated us on so many levels and these were the courageous men who led us to victory.

Edgar Mitchell became a fervent believer in UFOs. James Irvin of Apollo 15 left NASA to form a church. So did Charles Duke. In a documentary by David Sington, Gene Cernan, another astronaut to land on the moon, stated that he became a believer in something bigger than himself.

Mitchell is quoted as saying, "What I do remember is the awesome experience of recognizing the universe was not simply random happenstance." How can you not change when you see the fragile Earth rise above the horizon of the lunar surface? How can you not ponder your place in the vastness of space?

When he returned, Mitchell founded the Institute of Noetic Sciences. It is a nonprofit organization that sponsors research into "the potentials and powers of consciousness." Their website defines "Noetic" as inner knowing. The institute researches consciousness from three perspectives—first person, second person and third person. This means they look into individual consciousness, consciousness between people, and physiological correlates or consciousness such as mind-body healing. Clearly, Mitchell's travels helped him see the possibility of there being more to the world than we understand or see today.

I believe that all matter in the universe is recycled. The same elements that formed the universe from the beginning of time are in all our bodies. Therefore, we are all made up of exquisite stardust, and to stardust we will return. I think this comes from my Jewish faith in which we believe that the cycle of life and death is reflected in the statement "ashes to ashes and dust to dust." The beauty of our existence is seen in the simplicity of life while experiencing the complexity of our lives.

We have all experienced pain and suffering. We have all experienced loss. When I am struggling, during the darker times of my life, I have always found comfort in the belief that I am not alone. I feel that the universe gives us the tools we need to survive as long as we are open to receiving them. I believe that the energy surrounding my life is there to help me get through challenges and tribulations. I also believe that there are no coincidences—just opportunities to learn and love.

No one taught me this more than my father. Growing up, I watched how he navigated life. He is a Holocaust survivor. The tragedy he lived through could destroy any human's capacity for love and joy. He was interred in four concentration camps including Auschwitz and liberated from Buchenwald. Yet, he is man of honor, love and a believer in the fundamental goodness of others.

A particular story struck me. My dad played on a soccer team at one of the concentration camps Not only did the games entertain the guards, but they were also used in the Nazi's propaganda's attempt to convince American spy planes that nothing unsightly took place at the camps.

One day, a guard approached my father. He told him to go to work at a factory instead of showing up for the game. My father was surprised, but the guard said that the team would be put to death after the game. It seemed they had grown too malnourished to play, so the Nazis needed to field a new team for their pitiful rouse to be effective. My dad took the soldier's advice. That day, his team was killed. My father was the only survivor. My dad knew only how to fix his bike, yet he now was working in a factory pretending to know how to use a wrench. That one act from the guard saved his life.

What made that guard warn my father? He never knew for sure, but he clung to moments like that. When, in May 1945, the Allies defeated Germany, my father was at Buchenwald. The prisoners did not know what was happening. So, he hid in a sewage pipe and went two weeks with no food and little water. When the Americans found him, he weighed sixty pounds.

When I ask him how he survived something like that, he often refers back to the guard that saved him. He said that "anger and hatred are a disease of the soul and can lead to illness and death." He is a walking testament to his beliefs that love and the connection between people and even their environment can lead to a good life filled with wellness.

Through his suffering, he instilled in me at an early age the importance of connecting with people. He is always trying to see the good in others. My mother accused him of seeing the world through rose-colored glasses. Maybe he does. Perhaps that's the best way to see the world.

For me, that connection my father saw so clearly allows us to become more open to the gifts of the spirit. In bad times, we need others to help take some of the burden off our souls. I needed people with me when my mother was sick. As she neared death, my connection to the spiritual side of life became more and more important, as it does for many people facing that struggle.

Perhaps that connection started with my grandmother. I never met my maternal grandmother but heard many tales about her. Her name was Sarah—I was named after her. She came to the United States from Europe when she was a one-year-old child. She was known in her community as the "American Beauty" with her blue eyes and black hair. My parents were at her bedside the night before she died after a decade long battle against ovarian cancer. She had been in a coma for several days. All of a sudden, my grandmother opened her eyes and asked my mother how her "four" children were doing. My mother said, "I only have two children."

"No," Grandmother Sarah said. "You have four beautiful children."

At the time, my mom assumed my grandmother had been hallucinating. Over nine months later, my twin brother and I were born on Mother's Day to a mother who was also born on Mother's Day. No better present could be given on that special day.

I have learned a great deal about the human spirit by sharing my mother's journey as well. She was diagnosed with Stage 2 pancreatic cancer in March 2008. She did well on bi-monthly infusions of Gemcitabine and an occasional blood transfusion and pancreatic enzymes. She was determined to fight this disease and to not let it take over her life. In the summer of 2009, she required a stent to alleviate blockage due to stones in the common bile duct.

This was the start of a summer of medical events and complications often due to medical errors and negligence. Her medical teams only looked at her diagnosis and often overlooked her determination and will. I lived 1000 miles away and tried to help manage her care from afar, but it was difficult and challenging at best. I flew in when situations deteriorated and with the help of a few dedicated doctors and nurses and a strong-willed family, my mom would pull through. Now she was fighting a hospital acquired infection. The conflict inside me to help her as a doctor but also as a daughter tore my heart apart.

While I was on the way to the hospital on a sunny August morning, my mom's blood pressure dropped drastically and she went back into septic shock. She was put on medications to raise her pressure. When I arrived at the hospital, my father was leaving—not aware that this was happening. I got the news from the pulmonary fellow at the nurse's station before I went into her room.

I did not sleep the night before—I was up reading about spirituality, reincarnation, and beliefs of different religions about the soul. I was tormented by how my mom looked the day before and concerned that something catastrophic was going to happen. This morning, I knew that I wanted her to be without all the tubes and lines and to somehow wake up and eat a steak dinner even if that was the last thing she did—strange, I know, but I wanted her to have her dignity and life back.

A few minutes after I entered the room, she went into supra-ventricular tachycardia—a very fast heart beat and her blood pressure and oxygen levels were falling. I told the fellow that this was happening and the code team was called. At first, the nurse pushed me away and then the respiratory technician moved me to her right side. I held her hand as the team put ECG leads and paddles on her chest. Although she was semi-conscious, I told her that I loved her and to not be afraid and that her family was going to be okay. I told her doctors which medications she had responded to in the past and reviewed the monitors and the ECG strips. I saw that the room was filled with 10 people-all there to help her. The medications were not working so I just squeezed her hand tighter and kept telling her I loved her.

The oddest thing was that I noticed the fellow trying to lead his team and was impressed by his calm. I watched her nurse try to push meds and saw her concern and urgency. As I watched my mom's heart beat so fast—over 240 beats/minute—I wanted the nurse to calm her. I felt my mom's love and she gave me the strength to know what she needed—I was not afraid. As they were getting ready to sedate her and to shock her, I told them "no." The attending doctor asked me in a soft voice to repeat it and I told them not to shock her-they could continue with the meds. I could not have my mom's body tortured anymore. It was as if the night before, her presence helped me to help her. I was prepared at that moment for any outcome.

I have led many code teams and have never connected to the person that I was helping. I kept the emotional distance to do what I needed to do so there may have been a part of me that went to that place, but I would have shocked her by what I knew in my training. But my beautiful and strong mother taught me something else to do—I knew that it would be wrong to do that to her. In the worst moment of my life, my mother was there to help me. After I said "no," I leaned over and kissed her face and then began to cry. The nurse who had been so tough and distant with me before all of this had tears in her eyes. Someone on the team gave me a tissue since I was wiping my eyes on my sleeve. My mother was not just some patient in room 7, she was a woman who was loved and maybe this team finally understood that.

I asked for someone to call the clergy and to call my oldest sister. I did not want the rest of my family to drive knowing what was happening. For the next few minutes, her blood pressure was up and down and it was hard to ventilate her, but it improved as the meds kicked in. When my family came, I told them what happened. We just surrounded my mom telling her we loved her and hoping she heard what we were saying. When my dad came in, he sang a prayer to her in his melodic voice and she moved and slightly opened her eyes.

Our cantor arrived a few hours later and when he sang psalm 23, she opened her eyes and smiled. I think that she even tried to mouth the words. When I left the hospital at 10:30 pm that night, she looked like she was sleeping. She gave me an incredible gift that day and helped to heal me with a mother's love. This helped me to cope when we decided to take her off the ventilator at the close of Sabbath a few days later. I felt her spirit and her love with me every step of this painful journey.

My mother's entry into the medical system actually began two years before this event when she fell and fractured her hip. After enduring months of painful rehabilitation to walk again, she fell and fractured her other hip and shoulder as she was leaving the medical center. She developed pneumonia and her doctor did not want her to undergo surgery to repair her hip. He felt that she would not survive it, and it was more humane to give her morphine. She was then placed in a hospice for comfort care. After a week of semi-consciousness, she opened her eyes and told our family that she could not have her funeral on Sunday because the Denver Broncos would be in the play offs and no one would come to her funeral. At that point, we fought to get her back to the hospital. Amazingly, her labs were almost normal even after a week of near starvation and dehydration. I will never forget the look on the doctors' faces when they saw her again at the hospital.

In healthcare, there are those who only can focus on data and statistics. They are experts in the science of medicine, but cannot comprehend the art of medicine. It is the inner spirit, the faith and love that surround a patient that can also impact the health and well being of an individual. Time after time, my mother exemplified this principle, but so many of her doctors were closed off to seeing this new type of reality.

Right after she was diagnosed with pancreatic cancer, her primary care doctor who had dismissed her as all ready dead, told her in an angry tone that she should not get another CT scan because they were expensive and she had a fatal disease so there was no point. This was the same doctor who had put her in a hospice two years before. She had wanted another scan because she wanted to see how extensive the disease was for possible treatment options. She courageously told him that she was going to find another doctor; she was going to get this study; and she was going to fight this disease with everything that she had in her. She marched out of his office and never saw him again. After that visit, she had more studies and she did fight this disease with all her might.

She had another physician who treated her lung disease. He had taken care of her for years, treating her asthma and bronchitis. Her relationship with him was very important to her and she valued every word that he told her. I could never quite understand why she trusted him so much, but she did. He always told her that she had nine lives after she had "survived" the hospice incident—I think he had a renewed faith in her ability to survive and thrive. But he always underestimated the power of her spirit and the love that she had for her family which propelled her successfully through one medical crisis after another.

I recall one exchange that they had while she was in the intensive care unit during her final hospitalization.

He told her, "I don't think that you will survive this time."

She replied, "Well, what if I prove you wrong?!"

He responded, "You have done it before!"

That discussion gave her the fuel to fight for weeks until a severe hospital acquired infection set in. The last note that my mom wrote me was "Dr. Y. said that I am to die." I told her that he was not God and he did not know that. But I knew in my heart he had broken her spirit and her will to live. He took away the very medicine, the anecdote that kept her spirits high and her desire to persevere. We could never get it back after that. The power of his words was stronger than any antibiotic or drug. I am not sure that he would ever fully understand this, but it taught me a lesson that I will never forget. There is more to health than medications. There is more to life than our physical bodies. We are of mind, body and soul, and our health depends on us realizing and caring for all three.

GOVERNMENT AND SPIRITUALITY

When you open a discussion on spirituality and medicine, many in an audience may lose focus. It is a topic that involves intangibles, constructs that cannot often be seen, or heard, or even understood under the pretext of science today. Often, when someone is skeptical, I point out that the United States government is more open-minded to it than that. The federal government recognizes the importance of alternative or traditional medicine. In October 1998, Congress established the National Center for Complementary and Alternative Medicine (NCCAM) as a part of the National Institutes of Health.

The NCCAM is the lead agency when it comes to research on healthcare practices that are not considered conventional. Its mission is to:

• Explore complementary and alternative healing practices in the context of rigorous science.
• Train complementary and alternative medicine researchers.
• Disseminate authoritative information to the public and professionals.

They group complementary and alternative medicine into four "domains":

1. Mind-body medicine, including meditation, yoga, and practices associated with spirituality;
2. Biological based practices, largely the use of herbal or botanical products; selected compounds such as vitamins, minerals, and other molecules assumed to have therapeutic value; probiotics or strains of bacteria thought to be benign and to have healthful effects; and selected strict dietary regimens purported to improve health and well-being;
3. Manipulative and body based practices, exemplified by chiropractic and osteopathic manipulation and massage;
4. Energy medicine, involving the use of verifiable energy fields, such as electromagnetic radiation and sound, as well as biofields presumed to convey healing energies from master practitioner to patient.

NCCAM has sponsored clinical trials on a vast array of therapies that even included acupuncture, St. John's Wort, and shark cartilage. One study found that St. John's Wort is not effective in treating major depression. Another found that red clover, hops and chasteberry may help in treating menopause, but more work must be done to assess their safety. Yet, another found that tai chi increased immunity to shingles in adults over 60 years old.

Despite being sanctioned by the government, the NCCAM is not without its critics. Kimball Atwood published his feelings about NCCAM in 2003. He claims the office sprung from the perceived positive experience of two federal legislators. He goes on to accuse the office of being political, being more committed to pseudo science and complementary and alternative medicine (CAM) advocacy, and less committed to rigorous science. He points to the NCCAM's studies on distant healing and the "transfer of neural energies" as examples of how the office has lost its direction.

Any way you look at it, the fact that the NCCAM continues to get funding means that enough lawmakers feel its work is worthwhile. CAM will always have its detractors. The challenge is centered in the application of western techniques to study non-western modalities. At the same time, as even modern history shows, some types of alternative healing become amazingly popular. One such phenomenon was transcendental meditation.

TRANSCENDENTAL MEDITATION

Deepak Chopra trained as an endocrinologist, but he became a household name through his work on mind-body medicine. One of the practices he is best known for is transcendental meditation.

Transcendental meditation involves 20 minutes of meditation twice a day and allows the mind to "experience the source of thought." This is called a state of transcendental consciousness. The technique came from an "ancient Vedic tradition of enlightenment in India." Vedic refers to the Vedas, Sanskrit texts dating back to ancient India. Most are religious in nature and address a number of deities.

A plethora of scientific research has been conducted on transcendental meditation. In 1970, a study published in *Science* found that the state of the body during meditation is different from common states of consciousness. Researchers found significant differences in oxygen consumption and heart rate by recording measurements before, during and after meditation. In 2006, the *Archives of Internal Medicine* found that the technique could decrease blood pressure and insulin resistance, and stabilize the functioning of the autonomic nervous system in patients with coronary heart disease.

One of the most compelling findings came from a study published in the *American Journal of Cardiology* in 2005. Scientists evaluated the long-term effect of transcendental meditation on reducing stress and lengthening life span. Looking at older patients with high blood pressure, they found that those participating in meditation decreased their risk of "all-cause" mortality by 23 percent and cardiovascular mortality by 30 percent.

Not all studies ended with such favorable results. Researchers searched databases of existing clinical trials relating to transcendental meditation's affect on blood pressure. Of the studies that fit their criteria, all were found to have authors with some affiliation to the transcendental meditation organization which may indicate bias. They concluded that the studies published to date on the effect of meditation on blood pressure had "important methodological weaknesses."

Transcendental meditation is just one example of Eastern practices that have gained footing in the West. Many health practitioners attempt to treat not just the body, but the spirit as well. Charismatic healers such as Chopra are responsible in a large part for the spread of these practices. At the same time, people must also be looking for alternatives to conventional medicine.

While these practices may be beneficial to some people in treating aspects of their illness, I do not believe they are replacements for seeing your physician. I do believe that complementary therapy may be beneficial but all your healers need to be aware of all of the practices that you are using. This is important to get the best out of the healthcare that you are seeking and to minimize potentially dangerous side effects. I recall one patient who was using Chinese herbs to stimulate her immune system but she did not tell her family practice doctor who gave her a vaccine and she had a significant reaction to the shot.

THE MIND/BODY CONNECTION

Not all attempts to heal both the body and the spirit originate in the East. Rabbi Harold Kushner, the author of eight books, including *When Bad Things Happen to Good People* is another important source when considering the role of spirituality in medicine. In an interview with *Time* magazine, the Rabbi spoke on the power of prayer. Interestingly, he mentions a study that was done with two groups of hospital patients. People prayed for one group while no one prayed for the second group. The results, he said, showed no difference in recovery between the two.

At first glance, his seeming support of such a study is almost troubling. He goes on to say, "God's job is not to make sick people healthy. That's the doctor's job. God's job is to make sick people brave."

One set of researchers set out to determine if social support is important to the recovery of stroke victims. They looked at the effect of family support over a six month period on three rehabilitation variables—functional status, depression and social status. They found that high levels of family support were associated with "progressive improvement of functional status, mainly in severely impaired patients." Another study looked at what the social support of a spouse does for men recovering from coronary bypass surgery. They found married patients "who received more hospital support (defined by the number of spousal visits to the hospital) took less pain medication and recovered more quickly" then those receiving less support.

I definitely believe that the mind and the body are part of a symbiotic system. Ignoring the health of one will inevitably lead to problems for the other. Cultures around the world have seen that since the dawn of humanity. I saw it for myself when I visited Peru.

SHAMANISM

I had just finished trekking over several days in the Andes to get
to Machu Picchu —a magical and a breath-takingly beautiful site in
Peru. My friend and I were basically on our own with a porter during
most of the trek since our guide was trying to help a couple of climbers
who were not in shape to do this type of excursion. There comes a point
of no return on this trek and they had to get to the end with his help to
get transported back home. So, in mostly silence over a few days, we
arrived at a sundial on a mountaintop and looked down to see the ruins
of Machu Picchu. At first I was not sure where we were, but then it
quickly dawned on me that we had made it. A warm feeling of calm and
serenity surrounded us. For the first time in a week, I felt relaxed and
joyous and it was not due to a lack of oxygen or a climber's high. No, I
felt like the site emanated a peaceful energy which welcomed us.

After spending a day exploring this ancient community and
climbing the treacherous route of Winay Picchu, we were ready to move
on to the Amazon jungle. We flew to Iquitos—a small city by the river
and boarded a broken down boat with a guide to sail to our huts in the
rain forest. I was surprised by the narrowness of this muddy river and all
its tributaries—like capillaries off a main artery. Children were playing
and splashing in the water and I all I could think about was the piranha
and parasites that were in the river waiting to attack the next victim.
We arrived at our new home for the next few days—wooden huts on
stilts to protect us against the floods of a torrential downpour. To the
sounds of howler monkeys, we arrived. Shortly afterwards, we were
joining a small group to go find scorpions under leaves—a fun excursion
that in the United States I would never think of doing.

While I was checking the batteries in my camera and flashlight,
I was hit with a sudden chill that shook my body. I felt like I had entered
the Arctic rather than a humid, sweltering jungle. I could not get
warm—I put on my new llama wool jacket, my gloves, hat and hiking
boots and I still felt like I was in a freezer. Every muscle in my body
began to hurt. I thought it would pass and still went on the evening
outing to find scorpions. It was not hard to find them, but something
else found me as well. While on the flight to the Amazon, a cup of Coca-
Cola landed on my seat. So even though I had washed off the sugar

water and changed clothing, fire ants could sense it. I began to feel a biting sensation along my legs and it got worse with each movement. I ran back to the hut and with the light of a kerosene lamp, I took off my jeans and could see the long stream of ants on my legs. Someone ran to get me rubbing alcohol to try to neutralize the formic acid that was eating through my skin.

By that point, I was now sweating and shivering and did not even notice the pain. Perhaps, it was a small blessing. I just wanted to lie down and close my eyes. What seemed like hours later, I woke up and told my friend that it was morning and we needed to get going to catch the sunrise on the river. It had only been less than an hour since I put my head on the cot and I was now hallucinating. I knew that something was seriously wrong—I began to check my body for rose spots—broken blood vessels on the skin for signs of dengue fever. I knew that I had been bitten by mosquitoes on the trek but had been taking Mefloquine—an anti-malarial drug and thought that the incubation period was too short for the disease to present. I also knew that I was in trouble and needed medical care, but now I was in the middle of the jungle in the middle of the night. A flight to the Centers for Disease Control and Prevention (CDC) in Atlanta, Georgia was out of the question.

The only option I had was to see the village shaman. I was told that he was a wise man and he would know what to do. So I very gingerly put back on some new jeans and made my way to the boat to sail downstream to his hut. I was expecting a frail old man with many wrinkles and wearing a bamboo leaf skirt. Funny how these images pop into your mind when you are in a different world. He looked younger than I expected and his smile and kind eyes put me at ease. He touched my skin and looked into my eyes and asked me questions through our riverboat guide who spoke his dialect.

I went into a hut that had many animals including a sloth, several snakes in cages such as a boa constrictor, python and an anaconda that he released outside and let us pet. He prepared a concoction of herbs in a small glass. It looked like black syrup and had a putrid smell. Although there was part of me that wanted to try it, I couldn't do it. I knew that I was sick but then how was I to explain to colleagues back home about what I just drank if I didn't get better and needed western medical care? This message was shared with the shaman who again just smiled at me and he began to chant. I closed my eyes and tried to breathe slowly as his voice filled the hut, hoping that whatever he was doing would work.

I went back to my hut and fell quickly asleep. As the sun rose over the Amazon River, I awoke feeling great—more energy than I ever had since the beginning of the trip with no muscle or joint pain or fever. I was ready to begin my day. Now, I still don't know what caused my symptoms—perhaps it was due to Mefloquine toxicity and dehydration from my prior trek. But I do know I felt wonderful and the shaman may have helped me get there. What a blessing to experience in the middle of a jungle.

Shamanism is or has been present in most cultures spanning the Earth. At its simplest, it originates in our need to look beyond facts toward the complexities of life. Some groups rely on one person among them that they deem to be more in touch with the spiritual realm. The communities give these shamans "privileged status to attend to those groups' psychological and spiritual needs." Shamans claim to be in touch with things that the average person cannot feel, see or know. In essence, they are responsible for the spiritual wellbeing of a group of believers.

I did not go into my experience in Peru as a believer. As I said, I did not even agree to drink the shaman's "potion." When I felt better the next day, however, you can imagine how my perspective changed. Who knows what happened? Maybe the shaman healed me—it adds a touch of mystical joy to the whole experience. Perhaps his chanting helped to decrease the stress hormones in my body which enhanced my body's ability to heal itself. All I know is that I felt better.

In his article about the Western reaction to shamanism, Stanley Krippner came to the conclusion that someone's interpretation of shamanism probably says more about that person than the practice itself. I tend to agree, specifically from my own experience. As such, I believe that those communities still utilizing a shaman find a benefit in their guidance and spiritual expertise. If they did not, shamanism would vanish from the Earth, for without a following, the practice cannot truly exist. At the same time, I doubt someone totally closed-minded about shamanism, and spirituality in general would benefit from visiting one.

RELIGION AND MEDICINE

As the health care reform debate heated up, it was not surprising that Christian Scientists were also involved in the discussions. The Church lobbied for insurers to cover prayer as a form of healing. A senior Church official, Phil Davis, was quoted in an article appearing in the *Chicago Tribune* on November 1, 2009, as saying, "We are making the case for this, believing there is a connection between healthcare and spirituality."

Who can forget the highly publicized stories of parents refusing to get their sick children conventional medical care and instead relying on prayer to heal them? In two charged cases, children died. There was the Twitchell family whose infant child died of an intestinal obstruction. David and Ginger Twitchell were convicted of involuntary manslaughter when their two-year-old son, Robyn, died of an obstructed bowel. The parents received ten years probation and were ordered to provide regular medical exams for their surviving children.

Another case involved William and Christine Hermanson. They were charged in the death of their daughter, Amy, a diabetic, because they refused to provide her with insulin. They were charged and convicted of child abuse resulting in third-degree murder. They received four years suspended prison sentence on the murder conviction and fifteen years of probation. They appealed, but the verdict was upheld by the district court. When the case then went to the Florida Supreme court, the district court's ruling was overturned, stating that "a person of ordinary intelligence cannot be expected to understand the extent to which reliance on spiritual healing is permitted and the point at which this reliance constitutes a criminal offense."

If you look at these two cases, something stands out. There is no doubt that these parents have so much faith in traditional healing that they risked their children's lives. As a doctor, it is hard for me to imagine a parent withholding insulin from a diabetic child. What stand out most to me, though, are the sentences these parents received. In essence, both sets of parents received lengthy probation. The fact that juries did not send these parents to jail says something. Even in these tragic cases, the strength of faith and prayer, the spirituality of healing, cannot be totally vilified.

According to Christianscience.com, Christian Science is "based upon a set of spiritual principles—laws relating to the nature of God and His creation—that can be applied with expected, consistent results." It was founded by Mary Baker Eddy in the late 1800s after she suffered a spinal disease that western medicine could not cure. She turned to her faith and created a religion.

Now, Christian Scientists often rely on prayer over medication to heal illness. At the same time, they state that "Christian Science does not involve pleading with God to heal the sick and then accepting his will, good or bad." They feel that God's will for everyone is a long, healthy life.

If a Christian Scientist chooses spiritual healing, often they do not do it alone. There are Christian Science practitioners who are educated by an authorized Christian Science teacher. They offer patients treatment specific to a patient's need. In most cases, this involves bringing the patient closer to the idea that they were created perfectly by God. Most treatments are based on context found in Mary Baker Eddy's *Science and Health with Key to the Scriptures*.

Christian Scientists are not the only people refusing western medicine due to religious beliefs. Many Jehovah Witnesses refuse blood transfusions. According to a *New York Daily News* article, in 2006, Harry Morales, a Jehovah's Witness, was stabbed in the Bronx. Due to his religious beliefs, he refused a transfusion, even though he was told that in doing so, he risked death. Harry Morales died soon after. Interestingly, a jury acquitted the accused killer.

Maybe the jury blamed Morales, somewhat, for his own death. It is hard to say. At the same time, this story highlights the blurry line between our spirit and our body. Even the legal system seems to have difficulty assessing the role religion plays in medicine. My advice is to use both if that is what you seek. If you or a loved one is sick, go to the doctor. At the same time, seek whatever it is that soothes your spirit and provides support to your soul in troubled times.

SCIENCE AND FAITH

One of medicine's most prominent researchers and a Director of the National Institutes of Health, Dr. Francis Collins, provided a scientific look at the existence of God. Dr. Collins was the leader of the Human Genome Project. He created and led the BioLogos Foundation, a group committed to harmony between faith and science.

After a "free-thinking" upbringing, Dr. Collins labeled himself an agnostic while in college. As his scientific expertise grew, so did his doubt. In graduate school, he became an atheist, believing that "everything in the universe could be explained on the basis of equations and physical principles." When he changed course and attended medical school, his contact with patients exposed him to the spiritual side of health. He saw firsthand how patients leaned on faith, and how that faith gave them peace in a time of severe stresses and pain.

After being asked by a patient whether he believed in God, Dr. Collins decided to apply his scientific background toward determining the possible existence of something bigger. That endeavor led to his *New York Times* bestseller, *The Language of God*. By first arguing the existence of a Moral Law, Dr. Collins journey led him to studying the human genome. Of finding a connection to a "common ancestor," he wrote:

"Rather than unsettling, I found this elegant evidence of the relatedness of all living things an occasion of awe, and came to see this as the master plan of the same Almighty who caused the universe to come into being and set its physical parameters just precisely right to allow the creation of stars, planets, heavy elements, and life itself."

One of the most interesting discussions he shares revolves around the ethical use of genetic engineering. He offers that, although there is a hot argument about the moral implications of perfecting the human race, we are already doing that in many ways. He offers the examples of immunizations and music lessons both designed to improve the well-being of the individual. His discussion leads to the consideration of situations such as the use of human growth hormone for children with pituitary deficiencies. He compares that to the use of this hormone simply to increase a child's height for just cosmetic purposes.

As medicine advances, these types of questions will become more frequent and complicated. Already some parents who use in vitro fertilization are testing embryos for inherited disorders are being accused of playing God. The line between science and religion is blurring more and more every day. Decisions on these issues cannot ignore the connection. If they do, they are only considering half the problem, and then the best decisions are not possible.

MIRACLES

Most people you run into can tell you one story that happened to them or someone they knew that might be considered a medical miracle. Dr. Sanjay Gupta, a CNN medical correspondent published a book entitled *Cheating Death*. In it, he tells the story of a high school boy who is diagnosed with a rare brain tumor. After the initial surgery, it seemed he was cured, facing 1 of 1,000 odds of the cancer returning. However, after the surgery, he suffered awful nightmares and serious depression. A follow-up MRI showed four new tumors.

The boy, facing dire news from his doctors, found hope in religion. He prayed and, one night, saw a shooting star that he took as a harbinger from the heavens. As his condition worsened, the boy asked his father, who was not very spiritual, to gather people together and pray for him. They held the vigil in the hospital as the boy wanted to connect his faith to the healers fighting for his survival.

At this point, Gupta discusses the close tie between hospitals and churches. Most hospitals house some kind of chapel. He quotes a study that found "about half of Americans say they pray to help deal with medical conditions." Many studies have looked into prayer and healing. One examined whether patients want their doctors to talk about religion with them. Seventy-seven percent felt that doctors should consider their spiritual needs.

One week after the prayer vigil, the boy had an MRI. The tumors had disappeared. The patient attributed his recovery to the prayer of others. How could he not? Although research on the efficacy of such a claim is indeterminate, we have seen how the mind affects the body. Whether a higher power healed the boy, whether the boy's mind helped heal his body, or the chemotherapy he received worked above expectations, we will never know. What matters is that the boy survived, and in surviving, shared the connection of spirituality and health with everyone in his life.

During times of crisis, people often turn to prayer to help them handle or understand the situation that is before them. This was quite evident following the 2010 Earthquake in Haiti, the poorest country in the western hemisphere. Both in that country and abroad, groups congregated to pray and find comfort among each other. Perhaps through chanting and music, stress hormones were reduced and endorphins and oxytocin were released providing a stronger sense of well-being and calm. However, through this spontaneous outburst of prayer, they may have also connected to each other spiritually which may have helped as well.

Some Haitians believe in Voodoo which has a strong spiritual or supernatural component. The Voodoo religion is an import from Africa during the slave trade days. It has a fatalistic component and has been used by Haitian dictators to control the populace while covering up corruption. While most Haitians are Catholic, there is syncretism or a fusing of the two systems for many. As the situation in Haiti grew more dire following one the worst natural disasters in history, it was and will continue to be important that Haitians maintain a sense of control and hope. The role that Voodoo will play may not be useful in this situation—only time will tell.

In the midst of chaos and complete destruction in Haiti, there have been moments of joy and what one may identify as "miracles."

People had been pulled through the wreckage of demolished buildings over eleven days from the Earthquake. They had been imprisoned beneath concrete without access to food or water. Doctors have always thought that after seventy-two hours without water, few people can survive. What happened in Haiti has shown that the human spirit, faith in a higher power, and love for life can sustain a person in the midst of extraordinary odds. I recall some of my colleagues doubting my story that my mom survived hospice—going days without food and water. Now, no one can doubt that a person who has a will to live can endure unspeakable horrors. The world watched Haitians pulled out from buildings some singing in voices so strong that you never knew what type of hell they had endured. I have also been awed by the compassion and love that the Haitians have shown each other and what the world has shown them. Perhaps that is one of the greatest miracles from this catastrophe.

In an article published in the *Southern Medical Journal*, Robert Orr, M.D. looked into whether doctors believe in miracles. He cited a study done by the Jewish Theological Seminary that asked that question to over a thousand doctors. Seventy-four percent believed they occurred in the past, 73 percent believed they occur presently.

He went on to discuss what constitutes a miracle, including how loosely the word is used now. For example, some, perhaps in jest, pray for a miracle for their football team to win the Super Bowl. In providing his definition, he quotes C.S. Lewis, calling a miracle "an interference with Nature by supernatural power." The question is, however, what is "nature," and what is "supernatural." The existence of space, the Earth, even water, could be linked to a supernatural or divine source, and definitely could be considered natural.

It makes me consider how the Catholic Church canonizes saints. The process starts after the person's death. After looking at the candidate's life and holiness, they move onto the step of beatification. This requires the proof of one miracle, unless the person was martyred. A miracle, in this case, must come after the person's death, and happen to someone petitioning the person for divine intervention. Most of these miracles seem to be miraculous healings. Once again, it is clear to see how the supernatural, the spiritual, is so closely tied to healthcare; and how healthcare should be tied to spirituality as well.

* * *

When I was around ten years of age, I had a dream that my father was shot in the stomach. I remember waking up quite upset and running into my parents' bedroom to check on my dad. My parents were sleeping soundly, and I quickly went back to bed but knowing that I would not forget that dream. In the morning, I told my parents about it and they smiled and told me that my dad was actually going for a medical exam that day for his life insurance and not to worry. That night, my dad came home with a clean bill of health. We had dinner, my brother and I did our homework and we went to bed. I recall being awoken to the screams of my mother during the night. She found my father in a pool of blood in the bedroom. He was hemorrhaging—bleeding from his mouth from a perforated stomach ulcer which had never been diagnosed in him before. Was this just a coincidence or did I have a premonition? I prefer to think that I was given a gift, yet I was not sure what to do with it at the time.

My father was the focus of another mysterious event in my life. When I moved to Washington, D.C., I was very busy traveling around the globe as the medical advisor for the Office on Women's Health within the Department of Health and Human Services. One night while on the road, I had a dream that I was working in an intensive care unit. I was wearing my white coat and the rooms were all white and glowing with a bright white light. I came to one room and the male patient told me that he loved me very much and I told him the same. When I awoke, I remember thinking that it was quite odd that I would have this type of conversation with my patient. Yet, I felt this deep, pure love for him that I wanted to share. I then called and checked my voice mail messages on my home phone and heard my mother's panicked voice that my father was in the hospital and that his heart had stopped twice. She said that they were able to get him back, but he was going to need open heart surgery. Was the patient in my dreams my father again? Was it a premonition? Did my love help heal him? I choose to believe that the special bond that I have with my family transcends the material world and it was my father.

It has taken me years to fully appreciate this special part of our existence. It is the golden thread that weaves our experiences together. Without spirituality and faith and a belief that there is some energy, some universal link that connects all of us, life can only be experienced in three dimensions. As a child, I intuitively knew that we all had a "gift" to experience the world beyond our usual senses, but did not know how to name it or identify it. Yet, I have had several experiences from my childhood onward that have shaped my views of what is possible when one's heart and mind are open. Perhaps, my lineage—descending from my Romanian/Hungarian father's "gypsy heritage" or my maternal grandmother who envisioned the birth of my twin and me less than a year before we were born—explains why I see things the way I do.

Whatever we call it—intuition, clairvoyance, paranormal—there has always been an added dimension to how I see the world. It is not something that I often feel comfortable discussing in public because of the touchy-feely, fluffy, new-agey connotations associated with this, but I have come to accept it and let it refine my perspective. It provides me with a brilliant palette of colors to see a world that otherwise would seem gray or just plain black and white. I am a doctor, a researcher—a person who loves numbers, data and hard facts. To be open to something that I cannot exactly define or prove has been a challenge for me. Yet, I now feel delighted that the possibilities of what we are capable of experiencing and learning are endless. There is joy and not fear in my vision of the world.

I think that as we go through extraordinary events in our lives, we are given opportunities to grow and to learn. For some of us, it may take more difficult journeys to accomplish what our souls need for that development. But at the end of our journeys, lessons hopefully learned, we go back to dust and ashes in the physical realm releasing the energy that coursed throughout our physical bodies.

If we are truly stardust, celestial remnants from the beginning of time, than it would make sense that we go back to the pure energy that makes us what we are. In my physics class, I was taught that $e=mc^2$, or energy is equal to mass times the constant of light squared. (It takes a relative small amount of mass to produce energy.) So in that perspective, my thinking or cognitive brain has an easier time accepting that concept.

I have had many other multi-dimensional experiences in my life which I feel enhances my skills to care for others and to grow personally and professionally. It even complements my ability to take a scientific approach to life, but with an open heart and mind that something may also be out there, though we have not found the tools to measure it. We often say that there is an art and science to medicine. They do not have to conflict with each other. Rather our patients and my colleagues as healers can benefit from these extraordinary gifts that we possess but may choose not to open. Imagine the day when we feel confident in our ability to heal with the instruments from our material world as well as our spiritual energy that we all share from the beginning of creation.

In medical school, I studied physiology and pathology, exploring how the body worked and broke down to a point of disease. Our goal was to learn how to appreciate the fine balance between health and illness. Doctors are not often taught in medical school to look beneath the surface and to ask what they may not be able to measure. When we do rounds or report to other doctors, we share lab values, radiology reports and physical exam findings. Rarely, would we discuss the spirituality or faith or the unexplained phenomena that envelopes a person's life. The bottom line was that if you can't measure it, you can't report it. That type of approach misses stellar opportunities to add depth and richness to our lives. I choose to explore the stardust connection that will always enhance and enlighten my journey.

Stellar Questions:

What is the difference between religion, faith and spirituality?

According to *The Merriam-Webster Dictionary*, religion is defined as: the service and worship of God or the supernatural, or a personal set or institutionalized system of religious beliefs, attitudes and practices. Faith is defined as: allegiance to duty or a person or belief and trust in God. Spirituality is defined as: of or relating to sacred matters. These are definitions that we have relied on to explain our feelings and actions.

As for me, I see religion as a formalized entity where I can place some of my beliefs and actions within it. It provides continuity for my past and future. It gives me an organization which connects my life to a community which shares my cultural norms and history.

Faith for me is the belief of something outside the three dimensional world I live in. It provides me with a reason to have hope in times of despair. I have faith that the universe is generally good. When there is difficulty or a void—it will be filled, but maybe not in the way I anticipate. Faith is the elastic cord that connects me to other people and to the universe.

Spirituality is more nebulous. I believe our body houses our spirits. When our body expires, I do not believe the spirit does. It may find another body to come back in or reincarnates. Do I have physical evidence for this? I don't. Yet, it gives me comfort to believe in the concept that the spirit never dies. Once, I had dream about my mom a few months after she died. She was talking animatedly about the poor quality of healthcare that she received and wanted her family to share that information. I woke up smiling. To me, it conveyed that her spirit is still around us.

Why are children more spiritual than adults?

Many children grow up playing with invisible friends. Is it really make-believe? Could they be talking to the deceased? You can neither prove it nor disprove it, at least not within the laws of science that we currently understand.

Researchers looked at the spiritual needs of hospitalized children. About half of the children they surveyed reported spiritual needs relating to feeling anxious, coping with symptoms and relating to their parents. Although the conclusion of the report is that considerable improvement can be made to meeting the spiritual needs of children; interestingly, those surveyed felt that the hospital was providing 60 percent of "what they deemed as ideal spiritual care."

Clearly, children have a special tie to a world that adults rarely visit. Is that tie due to naivety or a purity of mind that eventually gets tarnished by the realities of an adult's life?

Is there evidence that Lourdes water can heal the sick?

In 1858, 14-year-old Bernadette Soubirous was out looking for firewood at the cliff of Massabielle near Lourdes, France, when she came to a grotto. There, she claimed a women dressed in white appeared to her. She returned home to tell her mother who forbade her to return. She went back three days later, and the lady appeared to Bernadette again. From there, more and more people accompanied Bernadette to the grotto to see the woman in white. A week later, she returned and the lady told her to dig in the Earth and drink at the spring. Bernadette dug in the mud and water bubbled up. By the next day, a spring had appeared. Bernadette and many others believed the lady to be the Virgin Mary, mother of Jesus.

Since then, the water at Lourdes is considered to have healing powers. In 1883, a French doctor, Baron de Saint-Maclou investigated those claiming to have been healed by the water. He was the first to have pilgrims produce medical certification of prior illness. In 1951, the International Medical Committee of Lourdes was established. Set up by the Bishop of Tarbes, it is the church's investigative body in charge of assessing the validity of healing claims by pilgrims. There are 25 members, ten of which hold "chairs in their medical schools."

According to the article in the *Journal of the Royal Society of Medicine*, about two million visitors to Lourdes have been registered as ill since 1858. Of those, 6,000 have claimed to be cured and 64 have been recognized as miraculous by the Catholic Church. From 1947 to 1977, an additional 27 have reached the level of investigation so that they have been deemed to be "medically inexplicable".

Although the method used by the Church to verify miraculous cures seems thorough, it is still hard to contribute the "miracle" just to the healing properties of the waters of Lourdes. Maybe the person's faith is the turning factor for them being healed. Who knows? Regardless, it is clear that there is enough interest and attention on Lourdes to merit it as a true example of how spirituality can be an important aspect of healing.

Do faith healers really exist?

People claiming to be faith healers definitely exist. The American Cancer Society defines the practice as, "the belief that certain people or places have the ability to cure and heal…through a close connection to a higher power." They go on to say that available research does not validate the practice. They admit, though, that it could help a patient's peace of mind and strengthen a patient's will to live.

Researchers studied child fatalities caused by religiously based neglect of medical care. They looked at 172 children who died under these circumstances and found that 140 children had a 90 percent chance of being healed by conventional or western medicine. An additional 18 had a greater than 50 percent survival rate. Their conclusion was that when faith healing is used alone, "the number of preventable child fatalities and the associated suffering are substantial and warrant public concern."

At the same time, prayer is obviously an important aspect of healthcare in the United States. In 2004, the National Center for Health Statistics and the National Center for Complementary and Alternative Medicine released a survey on American's use of alternative medicine. They found that 45 percent of Americans turned to prayer when facing health concerns and 25 percent asked others to pray for them.

I tend to believe that if one relies exclusively on faith healing, more harm can occur to the patient. Faith healing can complement conventional medicine as long as there are no large financial incentives for either modality.

What is the role of dreams?

No one can doubt the importance of sleep. We spend about a third of our lives doing it. During sleep, our bodies rest but our minds are at work. The brain is busy. It is creating new connections that help us learn; and it dreams.

Dreaming usually occurs about 90 minutes after you fall asleep during Rapid Eye Movement (REM). During this time, your muscles are "temporarily paralyzed so that they cannot act out any dreams." The study of dreams is called oneirology. In an interview with Discovery Health, dream expert Patricia Garfield described dreams as a "three story house." She said that basement is the body's physical response to dreams. The main floor is the aspects you sense visually, audibly and sometimes even through the sense of smell. The top floor, she said, there is something else. Whether spiritual or simply the creative mind at work, she says sometimes people dream of a loved one only to find upon waking that the person has passed away.

That brings us to near-death experiences. We hear the stories all the time. People pass away, see a bright light or feel a sense of calm, and then are revived.

In an article in the *Journal of Advanced Nursing*, researchers looked at the concept of the near-death experience. They concluded that so many people claim to have these experiences that nurses must be trained to deal with a patient who goes through a near-death experience.

Another study looked at near-death experiences in children. It reported that four out of seven children who survived cardiac arrest reported having an experience. The types included traveling in a tunnel, seeing beings dressed in white, and having a sense of being out of the body. This is an interesting study because it strengthens adult reports by lessening the chance that they are a construct of what we learn about death as we age.

Astral travel is another form of out of body experience that can occur during the dream state. It involves the existence of a body that can exist and travel outside our physical body. It travels along the astral plane, another dimension populated with spiritual beings. In Kabbalah, it is called the World of Yetzirah. In Islam, it is the Barzakh.

Clearly, dreaming has a practical purpose. It is a time for the mind to process memories and perhaps there is something more to them. Maybe it is an avenue to spiritually connect with loved ones as well.

Is there reincarnation?

Dr. Brian Weiss graduated from Columbia University and Yale Medical School and is the Chairman Emeritus of Psychiatry at the Mount Sinai Medical Center in Miami. He had a patient who told him of her journey through past lives. When he and other scientists evaluated her past life regression they validated the patient's memories as the facts fit. The experience changed his life. The therapist ended up learning from the patient.

Since then, he has seen many patients who have touched on lives they have lived or looked into the future. His work has made him a firm believer in reincarnation. I believe that all energy was created at the beginning of time. I think we are here to learn lessons from each other and we keep coming back to relearn and to teach others. Love doesn't die.

Have you ever noticed that there are some people that you feel more comfortable with and there are others that invoke distrust or anger for no particular reason. Could it be that you shared another life with them and are now reliving those past emotions? Many religions believe in reincarnation and people find comfort knowing that they may connect with a loved one again. Our opportunity for discovery in this area is as wide as the universe.

How does the Kabbalah relate to health?

Kabbalah is an aspect of Judaism that attempts to bridge the gap between God and humans. It is a discipline that adheres more to the mystical aspects of the religion. According to the Bnei Baruch Kabbalah Educational and Research Institute, it is a mystery only known to a few people, and often misunderstood by the rest of us. Kabbalah teaches the relationship between our universe and the "eternal and mysterious Creator." They go on to say that "all the world's forces descend from this comprehensive force (the Creator). Some of these forces are familiar to us, such as gravity or electricity, while there are forces of a higher order that act while remaining hidden to us."

The Zohar is the text that lays the foundation for Kabbalah. It outlines the four levels of interpretation: 1) Peshat, 2) Remez, 3) Derash, and 4) Sod. Peshat represents the most direct interpretation, Remez a more allegorical one, Derash a more imaginative one and Sod the most mysterious interpretation.

According to the Kabbalah Heritage Institute, Kabbalah spiritual healing is a practice using ancient "Kabbalistic spiritual techniques" to conduct distance healing. The idea is that they heal the soul, thus healing the body. They define the healing method as "an intentional distant mental influence process within the context of sacred Kabbalah through which the practitioner is able to have an effect on the physical and mental condition of their client."

Often, two Rabbis work together on a particular client. To heal the client, one practitioner accesses a higher level of consciousness. The other helps the patient on a more earthly plane. The practitioner in the altered state attempts to find the klipos—the adverse patterns within the patient—and tries to correct them.

Like any other alternative medical practice, I think it has its place. At the same time, it should be performed in conjunction with a conventional healer or doctor. Again, using complementary medicine may be the best route for you. It is your decision and should not be influenced by others such as celebrities who promote it for their own needs and attention.

What is the link between Alcoholics Anonymous and spirituality?

Alcoholics Anonymous (AA) defines itself as "a fellowship of men and women who share their experience, strength and hope with each other that they may solve their common problem and help others to recover from alcoholism." Step 2 of the group's *Twelve Steps* is, "Came to believe that a Power greater than ourselves could restore us to sanity." Step 12 is, "Having had a spiritual awakening as the result of these Steps, we tried to carry this message to alcoholics, and to practice these principles in all our affairs." Clearly, spirituality and God are a large part of the group's treatment.

In a commentary in the *American Journal of Psychiatry*, Marc Galanter, M.D. looked at the role of spirituality in Alcoholics Anonymous. After evaluating the research, he came to a familiar conclusion. Spiritual-based treatment can have a beneficial effect, but should be paired with conventional medical care as well. He also posits that it can be harmful if it causes conflict for the patient or keeps them from seeking help from a doctor or therapist. Many people have been helped with AA, and it is through their belief in a higher power that they are able to achieve sobriety and to help others.

CHAPTER NINE
BLOGS OF ADVICE
—www.BEWELL.com

When I began the journey to write this book, blogs, Twitter and text messages were not even a part of our vocabulary. Now we live in a world, where every second can be recorded. Perhaps this is an ideal way to connect all of us on this planet, and beyond to the outer reaches of our galaxy, but it can also leave us overwhelmed and inundated with too many stories, pictures, and commentaries.

I entered the 21st century of technology by writing my first blogs during the presidential campaign of 2008. It was eye opening to see how fast and widespread I could share my political views using this new medium. I enjoyed reading the responses and could not wait to write more. It was the start of my "addiction" to this form of communication.

During the campaign, I wrote editorials to several newspapers and blog sites—often on controversial topics such as reproductive health. I knew that I would stir the pot of discussion—some of which would be pretty aggressive and angry but at least there was a conversation in the safety of the Internet. When some of the discourse would get nasty, I would ask fellow campaigners and friends to join in to add some balance. I could sense the power of this technology to shape opinions and policy.

Shortly after the election in November 2008, a new health information website called www.BeWell.com was launched. I was the medical editor of several "communities" on this website including reproductive health, veterans' health, and aging and caregiving. All these issues that I am passionate about would become subjects of my blogs. I share a selection of them with you in this chapter. I now had an open forum to express my views and entertain questions. It was an ideal fix for a blog addict.

I began writing about everyday issues that I experienced in my world or saw in the news. I learned to choose wisely as I could write all the time and never get the rest of my work done. I wanted to share only viewpoints that I thought could serve a purpose and help educate. However as I wrote, I was learning more about my own core values and what I wanted in my life. In a way, I found that this doctor could heal herself through observation and awareness and sharing her findings with the world. Blogs became my starship to travel through the human community at warp speed!

It was not until I went through the travail of my mother's illness that I truly began to value what this website could do for others and for me. I began to write about some of the excruciating experiences of watching a loved one struggle and fight to stay alive. I also found it an ideal platform to share my views on sensitive issues facing our veterans and their families. On many occasions, people would contact me and thank me for sharing this very personal side of my life. My words became theirs. I think that this helped to provide comfort during some difficult moments. Fortunately, there were also exciting and joyous times to share as well—providing balance to this complex existence that we call life.

Life is filled with a series of adventures that are only made more fascinating and meaningful when experienced with others. Thank you for sharing this stellar journey through the universe of women's health with me.

* * *

Simple Steps You Can Take to Protect Your Health

I saw an interesting program on NBC's *Today* yesterday morning. It focused on actions one can take this month to help decrease taxes for 2008. With the market crashing and soaring around us, it was a timely topic. I felt quite pleased at the end of the show, since I completed many of the steps this past week that were mentioned, such as donating to charities, taking losses from the market, and keeping track of itemized expenses. It can all add up to some savings...which helps!

But it got me thinking about whether we have the same concern about protecting our health as we do with saving money. Too often we don't think about our health until we get sick. It is a natural response, but I think that it may not serve us well when we can take simple steps to stay healthy. I'd like to share with you some of the basic health tips that I give my patients around this time of year. Think of it as end-of-the-year advice to protect your health account.

Step 1: Make sure that you have made appointments for your physical exam and necessary screenings, like pap smears and mammography and pelvic exams. There is some debate about whether you need a complete physical; discuss this with your doctor. Even if you decide not to have a full physical, it can be a good time to discuss health issues and get advice on prevention strategies such as nutrition, physical activity, or smoking cessation.

Step 2: If your insurance deductible expires at year's end and starts anew, it may be economical for you to get your prescriptions filled now for the coming year, as well as any procedures.

Step 3: If going to a doctor is stressful, ask a friend or family member to come with you. A companion not only provides emotional support, but he or she can also ask questions you may forget or get you home safely if you're groggy from a procedure. You can also use the time for bonding and stress release after the appointment. Consider getting lunch, grabbing a tea, or doing a bit of shopping (a little something to look forward to after your appointment can take the edge off a sometimes-stressful event).

Step 4: If you have a test, ask when the results will be ready and how you should get the results. Ask if the doctor's office will call you or if you need to call them. You may also want to ask them to write down the tests that you undertook for your own files. This is a very important point and can make a big difference in your health! Don't assume that if you don't hear anything that everything is fine. I know from personal experience. My mother had been complaining of belly pain for over two years and was told that it was nothing. I did not know that she even had a CT scan over two years ago or I would have followed up on it. She was never given the results, so she assumed that nothing abnormal was seen on the scan. Unfortunately, there was something suspicious seen in the pancreas and the recommendation on the report was for follow-up studies. But no one followed up on the report. Last March, she again had more pain, was losing weight and had a high blood sugar level. She had another CT scan, but this time, a tumor in the pancreas that was very large and now inoperable was seen. The partnership between you and your doctor is an important one, and you need to make sure that you are informed of all your results.

Step 5: Keep your New Year's resolutions reasonable. It can be small steps that can make a huge difference.

The Gift of Time: Life in the Slow Lane

I had the privilege of speaking at the recent Massachusetts Governor's Conference on Women. Over 5,000 women came to hear talks about health, wellness, life balance, career development, and transitions. The sessions were lively and, at times, provocative.

One message that kept resonating throughout the sessions focused on time. We are so focused on the clock—with always too much to do and too little time to do it. One speaker mentioned that we are so obsessed with getting to our goals and final location "on time" that we often miss the exciting journey that takes us there.

How often do we not see the world around us because we are so focused on our final destination? I know that I do that. In fact, this trip was a fine example. I've been to Boston many, many times—to give lectures, visit hospitals, and interview for fellowships and jobs. Yet, I never really took the time to see the city—the neighborhoods, parks, restaurants, or really even the local residents.

This trip I tried to slow down and take it all in. (And it wasn't even the ice storm that swept through the Northeast while I was there that made me do this.) Since I was on my own, I took the opportunity to talk to everyone that I met—without reservation: the taxi drivers, waiters, women attending the conference, ticket folks behind the airport counters, hotel employees, and even fellow restaurant goers. It was a delight to listen to the various accents and hear so many different views and beliefs. Naturally, everyone had an interesting opinion about the state of the world!

One thing that I noticed is that as I slowed down to talk to people and simply observe, time seemed to slow down as well. I still got my work done, had time to get in a bit of exercise, check all my emails, and speak to my family. Yet I felt less stressed.

I guess this notion is what is meant by living in the moment and not focusing on the future. I still have many miles to go before I get this down pat. For example, I know that I want come back to Boston and explore—hopefully in the spring. But in the meantime, it feels great to just sit here in the airport and watch fellow travelers go by.

Live a Little This Holiday

I am often asked during the holiday season if it is possible to stay healthy and still enjoy all the delicious treats that are around us. The answer is a resounding "yes!" Just keep in mind that you don't have to eat everything that you see or is put on your plate. The sampler package may sometimes be the best way to go.

This week my colleagues and I at NASA had a dessert party after a lovely lunch out to celebrate the season. When we came back to the office, the conference table was filled with cakes, cookies, pies, and ice cream galore—enough sugar to keep everyone energized for the entire new year and probably enough calories too boot. Naturally my co-workers baked these delights, so it would have felt terribly rude not to imbibe. My solution? I put a small spoonful of each treat on a little plate, so I could taste and enjoy each dessert without feeling overindulgent. I call this conscious eating.

When it comes to most of life's simple pleasures, I don't believe in strict abstinence (unless, of course, there is a medical reason to completely refrain, such as alcoholism). Often when we abstain from something that we really want, we risk overdoing it if we finally get our hands on that "thing" and succumb to temptation. It's true for food, alcohol, shopping, sex, and other many other joys. Our brains are simply wired to increase levels of dopamine, which come with the indulgence. And those higher levels of dopamine give us a sense of well being. But you don't need to eat the whole pie, drink the entire bottle of wine, or buy thousands of dollars worth of clothes or electronic gadgets to achieve this sense of pleasure. A little bit can go a long way! Recent European studies have shown that just one glass of wine (two glasses for a man) can increase a woman's blood levels of omega-3 fatty acids, which in turn can improve heart health by reducing blood vessel inflammation, increase the "good" HDL cholesterol, and maybe even decrease blood clots.

So perhaps, in the words of on old song, "a teaspoon of sugar can make the world go around and around." It just doesn't need to make our waists grow with it!

Gift of Self: The Power of Volunteering

On Christmas day, I was part of a volunteer group that donated time to a women's shelter in my local area. For years, I have volunteered in various soup kitchens and shelters during the holidays, and throughout the years I've served as a volunteer doctor. On Wednesday, I went to the shelter not as a doctor, but as a member of the community.

The other volunteers and I gave presents, served cookies, played bingo, and talked to the women staying at the shelter. I wanted to know their stories. Some were very willing to share them, others were suspicious of my motives, and some simply did not want to talk. At first, when we all gathered into the small room that served as the dining room, play room, and living room, some of the women just stared at us (a small group of four volunteers), but by the time we left, we were all hugging, waving, and smiling at one another. It's amazing how, in just a few hours, the human connection could transform us all—perhaps just for that moment and maybe, for some, a longer period of time.

There was one woman from South America, wearing a colorful top and head covering, who said that she was supposed to be in this shelter for her spiritual growth; another who lost three of her five children in Africa; and a young woman from South Africa who dreamed of becoming a doctor and came to the U.S. for new opportunities, only now to have no place to call home. Some were very debilitated by their psychiatric illnesses and drug addictions; those women would occasionally join us and then drift away. I helped one woman, who could not talk, play bingo. She was in a wheelchair and had limited access to her hands. In order to eat her dessert cookies, she had to put her head to the table and grab the cookies with her mouth. We would put small buttons on the numbers on her bingo card and she yelped out when she won the game. Ironically, her present was a pair of gloves that she'd always need help putting on. But her smile was a priceless present to all of us volunteers.

This shelter is struggling to stay open and the people who work there day in and out are the kindest angels one could ever meet. Our new President-elect, Barack Obama, believes strongly in advocacy and community support. As we come into a new year, we will all be asked to participate in our community and to give a little bit of ourselves. We are all facing struggles and hardship, loss and grief, but sharing our time and our love can make the journey less lonely and sad. I promise you that the reward will be bigger than you can dream.

Nature's Gym

It was a treat to be able to do yoga and take a weight training class on New Year's Day. As I was leaving my house to walk over to the gym, I took a quick glance at my backyard and saw a mess of downed tree limbs and leaves scattered about—remnants of a lethal windstorm from the day before. I remember thinking, a bit forlornly, that I would again have more heavy yard work to do over the weekend. Although I like to garden during the warm days of spring and summer, winter forays do not bring a smile to my face.

At the end of my gym class, the instructor reminded us to be patient over the next few weeks, as the gym becomes more crowded with folks wanting to honor their new resolutions…at least for a short while. We all laughed at that notion—some commenting that resolutions were made to be broken. But it got me thinking that we tend to only recognize our excursions to the gym as the only way to get exercise. I guess there is a nice ritual to being a member of a fitness club: We change into our exercise gear, some even put on make-up (I'm just glad to wash my face and put on my favorite baseball cap), we chat with friends or warmly acknowledge familiar faces, and jointly share in the agony and bliss of a strenuous class.

Yes, there is a structure to that setting, but nature can also provide us with golden opportunities to improve our health and preserve well-being. Think about it: We can get aerobic exercise and even weight training to strengthen our muscles and bones when we rake leaves or shovel snow. The best part is that we get to be outside, taking deep breaths of fresh air and maybe even waving to our neighbors whom we may not see throughout the winter season, as we hibernate in our warm and cozy homes. There can also be a sense of accomplishment as you gaze out at a clean lawn or a safe passageway cleared of snow.

So come this Saturday, I vow to wear a smile on my face as I put on my hat, scarf, and gloves to visit the biggest gym around me: my own backyard!

Heart Health & Other Diseases of the Month

As we enter February, we are bombarded with articles and ads on heart disease. February has become "Heart Health in Women" month. Perhaps, Valentine's Day has something to do with it—all the lovely heart drawings on cards and candy have inspired a public health effort to encourage women, their families, and doctors to think about the number one killer of women in this country. The NIH and the American Heart Association have adopted the "red dress" as the symbol of heart health (I have wondered if men would get "red ties" as their symbol as a way to achieve gender equity since heart disease is the leading killer in men, as well). While it is good to have extra attention paid to important health issues, I hope that we can use it to galvanize a greater effort throughout the year and not just for the month.

Heart disease kills as many women as all the cancer deaths together. We know that women present with symptoms that are typical for women such as nausea, shortness of breath, weakness, and fatigue. Often a woman and even her doctor may not detect that these symptoms are associated with heart disease. Campaigns geared to women have helped to raise awareness, but still many don't know that heart disease is something they should think about and take action to prevent. Perhaps because breast cancer is so visible and it attacks such an intimate part of our bodies, the level of fear and concern has been so high. I don't want us to become a nation full of competing "diseases of the month." And so many of us have loved ones who are afflicted by several conditions—it is hard or almost impossible to rank which has priority. Perhaps one way to overcome this is to focus on wellness.

I recently attended a meeting of the new UN Council on Gender-based Health. This group has been convened to raise awareness of gender disparities in health across the lifespan and across the world— a very lofty task. During the first meeting, we raised the concern about only focusing on disease states and had some agreement that a focus on wellness may be a productive approach. So many of the chronic diseases that afflict women (and men) are based on behaviors that we can control or change, such as nutrition, physical activity, smoking, substance abuse, and even sleep and stress reduction. Of course, some of us live in environments that can be very dangerous and we know that poverty is perhaps the "greatest carcinogen." Yet, small changes in behavior can lead to huge advantages. Wouldn't it be interesting if instead of highlighting a specific disease during the month, we celebrated a positive behavior and ways that we can achieve it?

Again, simple steps lead to a longer and healthier life.

Caring for My Parents

I received a call from my sister last Friday night as I was heading out to have dinner with friends. She told me that she was on her way to the hospital in Denver, and that she had just called an ambulance for my mother who was found unresponsive at home. Naturally, feelings of sadness, helplessness and frustration poured over me.

This call was one that I have come to dread and, at times, even to expect. Last March my mom was diagnosed with pancreatic cancer. She has a trach to help her get oxygen into her lungs, as she has underlying chronic obstructive pulmonary disease, scar tissue from prior lung infections, and lives a mile high in Denver, where it's quite common to see folks walking around with oxygen tanks. The prior week my mom didn't seem her usual energetic and feisty self. I was concerned and talked to my family about it, but there was very little I could do. Over the past year, I've traveled back and forth to Denver very frequently—often putting out fires and trying to get my parents on a routine that's more stable and healthy. The period of calm or healthy new routine would last for about a week after I returned home to D.C. and then usually something awful would happen, like a fall or mistake in medication, which would require another hospitalization.

I have been trying to get my parents additional nursing assistance in their home, as my dad—who has been vigilantly caring for my mother—has diabetes and a heart condition. My parents have been a team for over 56 years: my mom cares for my dad and vice versa. They are both incredibly independent and love their privacy and routines. And often asked me to just be "a daughter" and not "a doctor." But I can't do it. Medicine is just wired into my DNA at this point. It's so hard to try to overlook dangers that I see lurking everywhere—slippery bathrooms, dust that causes breathing problems, unhealthy meals, medications covering countertops (some quite outdated), and narrow hallways that can trap oxygen chords and cause falls. The list could go on. Yet, this has been their home for almost 40 years and is their place of peace and security.

I have wanted home assistance if they would not move to assisted living, but that had been vetoed as well for various reasons. I've tried to learn how to "let go" and let my parents live the life that they choose...even if would not be my path. Perhaps the lesson in all of this is that we can still love and care, but know that we each have to make our own decisions. It is not like a parent caring for a child, but perhaps the same love and concern are there. Every day, I have to remind myself of that lesson. It is such a difficult one.

Welcome Back, Science

I waited eight long years for this week. I remember the August night in 2001 when the nation was told that stem cell research would be severely curtailed. Weeks later we learned that many of the stem cell lines that we could use were contaminated. During that time, my former office at The Department of Health and Human Services was also told to create embryo "adoption" programs, not "donation" programs. We were also getting reports that scientists were being blocked from using scientific evidence to guide policy. I remember being unable to publish unless I went through extensive review by the Department. It often took more time for that process than for the peer-reviewed one. We could not talk about contraception or sex education and needed to advocate on behalf of abstinence. The list of the attack against science was long. I finally resigned my position that I so loved in August of 2006. It was just too painful to do my job when the environment no longer supported science.

This week, President Obama signed an Executive Order allowing research on stem cells and for the National Institutes of Health to guide the policy. He also signed a memorandum protecting the scientific process from politics—letting policy be guided by science, not faith nor ideology. During the election, I wrote about this process in an editorial for the Rocky Mountain News in Colorado. I received many responses to my editorial—often many of them angry and a bit scary. Yet, even though it made me uncomfortable to receive these hostile comments, I was glad to see the dialogue. For too long, we were not sharing our views. I wanted to wake up folks and help them take a stand. I don't know if it changed anyone's views, but maybe some input from the other side was heard.

I have been to several meetings at the NIH and NASA recently and there is definitely a different spirit in the air—one of optimism and hope. Finally to have science back in our hearts, minds and the budget allows us to dream of new solutions and answers to the questions and issues that will help make our lives healthier and longer.

Be well!

Art Imitating Life

I arrived in New York City yesterday afternoon for a meeting of the UN Council on Gender-Based Health at the United Nations. As luck would have it, my hotel was next to the Eugene O'Neill theatre and one block from TKTS, the ticket discounter for Broadway and Off-Broadway shows. I walked the one block and discovered that the play "33 Variations" starring Jane Fonda was available for half price and, conveniently, it was at the O'Neill theatre. What a great coincidence!

The show was listed as a musical, which I was delighted to see. I've been working non-stop—taking care of ill family members, writing a book and articles, and renovating a kitchen with a contractor who forgets to show up—so I was more than ready for a relaxing time-out. I didn't know what the show was about, but knew it got great reviews, so

I bought a ticket. Fifteen minutes later I was in my first-row, center seat. Amazing how everything worked out.

When Ms. Fonda entered the stage, the theater erupted with applause. I couldn't believe how close I was to the actors. I could see every little detail of Ms. Fonda's expressions, including her delicate hands and the color of her nail polish (things only a woman would really notice and appreciate). For the first 10 minutes, I was in bliss.

Then the story evolved. As it turned out, "33 Variations" is a show about a music professor who has been diagnosed with amyotrophic lateral sclerosis (ALS). It explores the protagonist's desire to complete her last book on Beethoven, as well as her reluctance to navigate the turbulent waters of her relationship with her daughter. What exquisite irony that, of all the shows on Broadway, this was the one I was attending...and not only that, but situated smack dab in the front row with the lights shining on my face.

You see, this was a story that resonated all to well with my own life. I've written about my mother's journey—our journey—through the world of pancreatic cancer. It has been almost one year to the day that she was diagnosed. Her brave fight, grace, humor, and travails have been a major part of my and my family's life. It was unbelievable to see a similar story play out in front of me.

During the intermission I called my mom to tell her I was at the show. She's still in a nursing/rehab facility from her last hospitalization from a month ago. She told me that the results of her most recent tests, which unfortunately revealed that her tumor was now pressing on her stomach and she would need another stent. It took everything in me to go back to my seat after that news.

Of course, the second half was filled with poignant details of the character's demise and eventual paralysis, as well as an evolution in her relationship with her daughter. I could hear all around me sniffles of quiet crying. It was like watching my life play out on the stage. Jane Fonda and her co-stars did a brilliant job. I could not stop my own tears from gently falling down my cheeks and tried to gracefully wipe them away. It was an odd experience. At times I felt that I was on stage, since I was so close...yet I was so alone. The saving grace is that there were wonderfully healing lessons expressed in the screenplay.

I do think that the universe does give us gifts when we most need them. This was one that I definitely did not expect. I know that it will take some time to appreciate it, but it will be valued.

Voices for Our Loved Ones: A Lesson in Health Advocacy

Last week I did something that I've never done before: I walked the halls of Congress, talking to Senators, Representatives, and their staff members from the states of Colorado, Indiana, and the District of Columbia. I've been to Capitol Hill many times over the years. In fact, my office is just a few blocks away. I've even given speeches in the Capitol Rotunda and in many congressional office buildings during hearings and briefings. What made yesterday different is that I went as an advocate for my mother and family—not in my professional capacity—to talk about an issue that does not have many voices: pancreatic cancer.

Pancreatic cancer is the most lethal cancer and yet it has the lowest amount of funding. 75% of those diagnosed with pancreatic cancer will not live past the first year, and the five-year mortality is less than 5%. Over 500 folks from across the United States came to Washington this week to talk to their congressional members about the disease that has devastated so many lives. From this group, there were only 40 survivors in attendance. Those who are battling this disease don't usually have the strength to come and fight for more funding and awareness. They can't run in 10K races or march down city blocks. They are valiantly fighting to stay alive—many trying anything that has a sliver of a chance to help them do just that.

When my mother was diagnosed in March of 2008 (yes, she is a fighter!), she asked me why it had to be pancreatic cancer and not breast cancer…because for the latter at least she'd have some options for treatment. It broke my heart to know that she was right. Because her mass was initially misdiagnosed, it was too late for surgery and there was very little to offer in regards to chemotherapy. Still, every week—and now every other week—she goes to get chemo, which has left her arms bruised from all the infusions. With strength and dignity, she is fighting this disease and refusing to give up…just like so many others who were also represented by their families and friends this week. We were their voices.

Although our group of family "ambassadors" was comprised of complete strangers, we were warmly hugging each other farewell after our second day together. It was as if we had known each other for years, bonded by a common history and shared pain. Amazingly, we spoke as a united team during each meeting even though we didn't practice.

Some things in life just work out that way when there is a common purpose. As a result, the message gets amplified.

There needs to be increased support for physician and patient education. Pancreatic cancer is not a "silent" disease. It is just ignored, since the symptoms are similar to other common ailments. We need more studies to help develop a screening tool—just like we use for breast and colon cancer—for more treatment options and perhaps even ways to prevent the disease. My mom's cancer grew out of a benign cyst in her pancreas. It was ignored by her doctor who never told her she had it. We have all heard about Justice Ginsburg's recent cancer diagnosis, which was caught because of strict surveillance for her history of colon cancer. Doesn't everyone deserve that level of care?

I am also concerned that the toxins in our environment may be related to this cancer, as well. Oddly, there have been four cases of pancreatic cancer diagnosed within a block of my parent's home in Denver over the last two years. For a disease that has an incidence of 38,000 cases per year (and 35,000 deaths), one needs to think about a link.

At the end of our meetings yesterday on Capital Hill, we all felt better because we had taken action over a disease that leaves us feeing impotent. It was also a reminder that we have an incredible gift as Americans: the freedom and responsibility to be a part of our government ('of the people, by the people, for the people'). Last week's efforts were for the people who needed our voices the most.

The Heart of the Capital

On April 28, 2009, Sojourner Truth arrived at the U.S. Capitol when she became the first African American woman to be honored among the statues. Her journey as a slave, an abolitionist, a suffragette, a speaker, and a writer was arduous and painful. Yet, through her words and actions she inspired a nation. Over 1,000 people—mostly women—gathered in Emancipation Hall, which houses the National Statuary Hall Collection in the new Capital Visitor Center. There, in that august room, we came to celebrate a woman whose life changed the way women were ultimately treated in this country and the rights that they deserved.

The soaring speeches by our congressional leadership, new Secretary of State, and the First Lady, along with songs and readings by children and celebrities, illuminated this extraordinary day. After the various tributes, the bronze bust of Sojourner Truth, who was six feet tall in her day, was unveiled. I, like so many of in the audience, remembered studying the "Ain't I a Woman" monologue in school, and it created a special feeling of kinship with the honoree.

As we celebrate Mother's Day, which is a very special day in my family, as my mom and my twin brother and I were born on that day, I recall the impact our mother had on our lives. Sojourner Truth, who bore 13 children and inspired generations to come, had some of her descendants at the event. Through congressional language and private funding, her descendants and the millions who come to visit the Capitol can now see that our nation was built on the shoulders of many who dared to be brave and fearless.

Following the event, I attended a congressional luncheon where I had to take care of guest who collapsed from a possible heart attack. Following that, I went back to my NASA office and faced public health issues surrounding the H1N1 influenza (commonly known as swine flu). Talk about a day filled with many highs and lows.

Later that evening I attended a lecture at the National Geographic Museum about the treasures found in the caves in the remote Himalayan kingdom of Mustang. Peter Athans, the world renowned climber who explored these caves, which provided insights into the beginning of Buddhism, said that it is through adversity that the soul grows. Sojourner Truth's journey towards truth and opportunity was a wonderful reflection of that concept. I have a new appreciation for my own journey and hope that you do as well.

No Time to Wait: Tackling the Physician Shortage

Have you ever had to wait to see a doctor? Perhaps it took you a few months to get an appointment or maybe you had to sit for a long time in a waiting room? When you are ill or not feeling well, minutes can feel like hours and months can feel like years.

Now imagine this: toss in another 46 million additional Americans wanting appointments with the same number of doctors currently in practice. That is just one scenario that could play out if we do not make dramatic changes to our medical workforce.

The American Academy of Family Practice predicts there may be a shortage of 40,000 family doctors in just 10 years if medical schools continue to graduate only half the needed numbers into primary care. It is estimated that by 2025, we will be short 124,000 doctors. There are already over 215 million primary care visits scheduled each year. Just think how many more will occur as the population swells and ages.

It is not just the patients who feel frustrated by the physician shortage; doctors feel the strain, too. Consider the doctors working in underserved urban poor and rural communities who want to retire or reduce their hours to part time and cannot without leaving a further hole in local care. We've all heard reports of some communities without any medical care whatsoever and patients who have to drive for hours to get it. I remember when I was a resident at the VA Hospital in San Francisco and saw patients who had driven five hours from Redding, California, to visit our clinics, including one patient who had just had a heart attack!

I always like to believe that by facing big challenges, we can grow and create exciting opportunities. Now is such a time if we dare to be bold and innovative. It's up to us to change the healthcare landscape in our nation. I want to share one solution with you.

At the turn of this century, I chaired the National Task Force on Physician Reentry when I was with the Office on Women's Health within the Department of Health and Human Services. At the time I wanted to examine reentry issues because I was contacted by so many fellow female doctors eager to return to practice after having raised their children. Initially I thought this was really just a women's issue. I was surprised to learn that men wanted the ability to have periods of clinical inactivity and then return to the workforce, too. Talk about an equal opportunity issue! The task force met for over a year and we published our recommendations in 2002 (Mark, S., Gupta, J. Reentry into Clinical Practice. JAMA. 2002; 1091-1096).

We all know that with the aging of the population the prospect of vastly expanded medical coverage and the potential need for increased numbers of doctors during public health emergencies such as pandemics, natural disasters, and bio-terrorism, immediate action is needed. For example, we see in Argentina that they have declared a public health emergency because their medical system is overwhelmed with the number of H1N1 (swine) flu cases that have occurred during their winter flu season. This could happen in the U.S., as well. Even though we are planning for it, we still need doctors—and lots of them—if the pandemic continues in waves over many months or years.

One potential solution is the development and support of physician reentry programs. Physician reentry is defined as returning to professional activity/clinical practice for which one has been trained or certified after an extended period of time. The Physician Reentry into Workforce project, established in 2006 and building upon the work of my original task force is a collaboration of over 20 physician membership organizations, regulatory groups, and educators.

Under the leadership of the American Academy of Pediatrics and the American Medical Association, significant progress has been made by this project to address competency assessment, educational, licensing, and credentialing requirement, along with strategies to encourage physicians to reenter clinical practice.

Although it is important to ensure that new physicians enter primary care, it would be a waste to not utilize the vast talent and rich experience of doctors who have left clinical practice but now wish to return to serve the public. We cannot afford to wait to build the pipeline of new talent.

If you believe that this is a good idea, please contact me or the White House (www.whitehouse.gov). It is through public support that we can change our healthcare system. There is "no time to wait." Our lives depend on it.

Updates from the Field: The Latest on H1N1

I want to share with you some updates I've provided to the various organizations and agencies I advise regarding novel H1N1 flu, commonly known as swine flu. Keep in mind that this is an evolving situation and what we know now may change.

1) Federal supervision of the novel H1N1 vaccine will be administered by public health departments to ensure strict oversight of the vaccine and its possible side effects. During a recent White House Summit, there was an announcement from the Centers for Disease Control and Prevention (CDC) about using other facilities, like health clinics, community centers, and schools as vaccination sites. Essentially, schools will try to stay open. The decision to close schools will take place at a local level where officials can weigh all the factors, including how many students and teachers are ill or whether or not certain schools have special issues, like a large population of students with special health needs. Private providers and clinics will be able to administer the vaccine so long as the clinics sign and comply with the provider pre-registration process/agreements, ensuring that the vaccine will be stored properly and administered according to standards and priorities. The VARS—an electronic system monitored by the CDC and state public health departments which tracks side effects—will be used. Additionally, there will be an electronic registry to monitor doses given.

It is estimated that schools may get the H1N1 vaccine for their students by the end of September.

2) The CDC will be conducting prospective studies to evaluate post-vaccine side effects and efficacy. For example, four sites around the nation will do comprehensive review, including evaluating at least 900 pregnant women and their use of over-the-counter medicines.

3) There are new treatment and prevention guidelines for pregnant women, who are four times more likely to have complications from H1N1 infection compared to the general population. It is recommended that Tamiflu (five days) be given for treatment or Relenza (10 days) be used preventatively to treat expectant moms. Relenza is inhaled and results in decreased systemic absorption, which may have a lesser impact on the fetus. (For those with asthma, caution is necessary when taking Relenza.)

4) If one presents with flu-like symptoms during the summer season, it is assumed to be novel H1N1 infection and should be treated. It is unusual for the seasonal flu to appear during the summer, but the H1N1 virus has done just that throughout the world. Studies now show that the rapid detection tests used to diagnose H1N1 infection are not accurate. The nasopharyngeal swabs using PCR-Polymerase Chain Reaction technology are recommended if there is concern about diagnosing and treating the infection.

5) New studies coming out of the United Kingdom indicate that children may experience more side effects to Tamiflu than adults, including vomiting, nausea, diarrhea, dehydration, and neuropsychiatric complications (nightmares, insomnia, and poor concentration). These side effects may outweigh the benefits, so more investigation is needed.

6) It is highly recommended that health clinics use separate rooms to isolate those suspected with H1N1 infection. Many believe it may even be wise to have patients with flu-like symptoms call in advance of arriving at health facilities, so steps can be taken to limit their exposure to non-infected patients. Those suspected to be infected with novel H1N1 should wear facemasks to prevent spread to others. Emergency rooms and even clinics may end up being the new incubators of this disease.

7) There is much debate over the strategy of removing pregnant women from working with suspected or infected patients. There are challenges to this approach, including an already limited workforce supply and the fact that some women don't even know when they are pregnant. Some have even suggested that this tactic may also be

appropriate for other high risk groups, such as those who are obese. This is not a very practical solution, but the need for it should be considered over time.

8) Seasonal flu vaccines are being shipped to the U.S. market and novel H1N1 studies are now ongoing at eight sites. I have some concerns about the H1N1 vaccines and their impact on the immune system. Some of my concerns, which may not be fully evaluated during these studies due to a lack of time, include:

- Impact of one's sex on response to the vaccine, as well as the use of adjuvant therapies on dosage. It's believed that the female immune and inflammatory response may be more robust, so perhaps women may need a smaller dosage. Might a smaller dosage decrease the side effects that some women experienced when vaccinated?
- Is there a higher risk for complications if one receives the seasonal flu vaccine and then is exposed to pandemic flu or given the first shot of pandemic flu vaccine? Will there be a cytokine storm (a serious immune reaction), since there is some cross over in the antigenic determinants and the immune and inflammatory systems will be activated?
- Is there a higher risk for complications due to cytokine storm if one gets the pandemic flu vaccine and then is exposed to seasonal flu or the seasonal flu vaccine?
- Will there be populations were the pandemic flu vaccine may not be effective?
- Will there be any impact if one gets one pandemic flu vaccine from one drug maker than another—such as those who travel overseas and get vaccinated?

Tight surveillance for side effects and efficacy will be essential as the immunization effort gets underway. Public service announcements have been funded and will appear now and throughout the year to help educate the public.

While the novel H1N1 presents serious concerns, it's good to keep in mind that the U.S. has developed a robust public health system over the years, which will help to protect our health and wellbeing. For most of us, what's key to remember is that if you do not feel well and have flu-like symptoms, stay home! There is simply no need to risk infecting others or to worsen your own recovery. A tincture of time, rest, and fluids is often the best medicine. If you're not doing well, call your doctor immediately. Keep in mind that your local emergency room may not necessarily be the best place to spend time.

Always stay informed and never hesitate to ask questions!

A New Year of "Firsts"

I came back to Denver this week to be home with my family for the first Rosh Hashanah or the Jewish New Year without my mom. It has been a week filled with sadness, tears, occasional laughter as we remembered stories from the past, and a desire to continue the traditions that my mom instilled within all of us. The first night of the holiday was sober and difficult. It was hard to believe that she was not there conducting the orchestra, which included all my siblings, to ensure that the dinner was served properly and in the style to which my father had grown accustomed.

We failed, even though we thought we had it all planned out, we could not get the dinner right. It started out with my sister asking who was going to sit in my mom's chair. You see, I had set the table and until my sister asked that question, I did not realize that I set a place setting for my mom. When she mentioned it, it dawned on me what I had done. I was in charge of setting the dining table for decades of holiday dinners and I always made sure that I set my mom's chair in the right place...nearest to the kitchen. I unconsciously did it again. Next, the chicken soup was cold, the matzah balls were cold, the glass holding the Sabbath candle cracked during the middle of the dinner and my sister's dog kept running around the house looking for her favorite person, my mom. Finally, she settled down when we put her on my mom's blanket on the carpet next to the table. The dinner was saved many times that night by the microwave oven.

I have been told by many folks that this will be a year of "firsts." My mom loved holidays and we centered our lives around them. Now, I wish that they would disappear because they make our loss more monumental, quieter and lonelier. I know this feeling will eventually disappear and we will have a year of new memories and, hopefully, a year filled with old traditions. My mom would love that.

What Does It Mean To Be a Cancer Survivor?

Last October I gave a series of lectures in Panama City, which was completely adorned with pink ribbons. The former First Lady of Panama was a patron for the breast cancer community, and through her support every major landmark and building was wrapped in pink. There was literally a pink ribbon everywhere you looked, adorning the airport, the shopping centers, the presidential palace, and even the Panama Canal. It was a wonderful way to raise awareness of a disease that affects over one in eight women over their lifetime.

Every October, we see this same level of enthusiasm in cities across America, which hopefully translates into more women getting their mammograms and feeling, connected to their bodies and their medical communities. A disease that for so long had been silent and associated with stigma has finally found its voice and its power base.

With more women surviving breast cancer than ever before, we now have an "army" of women to help raise funds for research and education. Often the best salve or medication for one who has experienced a life altering or life threatening illness is the ability to help others facing a similar situation. But how does one define being a survivor? Is a survivor someone who has gone through chemotherapy, surgery, and/or radiation and is still able to get up in the morning and face the new day? Is a survivor someone who has been disease free for a year, five years, or 10 or more years? Or is a survivor someone who has faced multiple bouts of cancer and yet still has a hope and indefatigable desire to live?

I never really thought much about these questions until a few months ago when I went cross-country skiing with my friend. She was diagnosed with breast cancer five years ago and endured the ordeal of chemotherapy. This past winter, she was diagnosed with metastatic breast cancer after doctors found tiny spots on her lungs. As we were gliding along a winding trail, she said she was sad that she could no longer call herself a survivor. While she doesn't feel ill and is able to do all the activities she did before this new diagnosis, she now fell into a new category: "a patient with incurable cancer." My friend still feels like a survivor, though, and has found joy and peace in her life. She has a desire to help the world through her spiritual training and doesn't want to be thought of as a terminal case...someone who was not a survivor.

Watching my friend and others navigate the challenging path of incurable cancer got me thinking about what it means to be a survivor. Like many, I followed Senator Ted Kennedy's valiant struggle to continue serving his country until the very end of his life despite having a brain tumor. (I will always be grateful to him for his support of an important piece of legislation to provide mental healthcare for our troops this past June 2009). We all watched in awe as Patrick Swayze, battling Stage 4 pancreatic cancer, not only starred in a television series, but wrote a book and spoke publicly about pancreatic cancer. My mother, who also fought pancreatic cancer, felt like she had a brother in him during her journey to combat the disease. (She did not die from pancreatic cancer, but from medical errors leading to a hospital-acquired infection). She also never gave up hope and continued to care for her family and community with her audacious sense of humor and honesty. She served as my editor for some of my articles and even for my new book, which will be published this coming year.

All of these men and women are survivors! They lived their lives fully and with a sense of purpose. They never gave up and they never gave in. Although they may always be associated with the cancer that infiltrated their lives, they survived it to be champions for those they loved and served. Their legacies live on.

A Time for Reflection

What a year! To say it was a roller coaster does not do it justice. I know that for many of us, the journey was filled with love, excitement and adventure but to balance it out add a touch of sadness, grief, and pain. Perhaps that is the path that we all need to take to appreciate what we have, to grow, and to fully feel the emotions of life. As I finish the last of my travel for the year, I now have a few minutes up in the air to look down on our beautiful planet and take stock of what has just happened. The promise of a new year provides us this ideal incentive to reflect.

There is a new movie called "Up in the Air"—the acting is superb but the story line is disturbing to me on so many fronts. I recently saw this movie and it made me think long and hard about my life. Some of the similarities to the main characters hit home—always on the move and planning my life around the next flight or train ride or even bus ride. Trying to balance home, family, work and self time—the simple things like getting some exercise or having food in my refrigerator or watering my plants always a challenge to accomplish. It is the most basic of activities that we all take for granted until we have to be organized to get them done. It makes me laugh when I hear my voice mail messages and friends have been trained to say "Wherever you are, when you get this message, give me a call."

I had a year that never slowed down nor provided many moments of peace and quiet. I lost my mom this year and I was with her throughout her battle to live. She cherished every minute. One of my favorite "moments of tranquility" was when I took her outside the medical facility and we sat in the sun for a few minutes—her face looking up, her eyes closed, her mouth in a smile—just savoring the warmth on her skin and the joy of being with her daughter. Yes this was quite a year—I was in Berlin for the fall of the Wall celebration, in New York to see an award winning play, on the Mall in Washington, D.C. to witness the inauguration of our new President, on Capitol Hill to speak about veterans' health and many other extraordinary events, but it was that moment with my mom that I treasure the most.

Next year, I promise to close my eyes and smile while the sun warms my skin and my heart. And it will be for more than one moment in time.

Help for Haiti

Another disaster has struck the planet—a natural disaster worsened by a manmade calamity. A 7.0 Earthquake struck Haiti yesterday, January 12. Thousands or perhaps even hundreds of thousands of people may have been killed, millions displaced and a capital destroyed. We have, in some ways, become immune to seeing or reading about these events—from the tsunami in Indonesia, the hurricanes and floods in the American South, and to the Earthquakes in Asia. Each year brings more names to a growing list that the planet is turbulent and volatile, and we are just temporary residents often living under conditions that are not conducive to surviving these events. We live too close to fault lines or shores, we build homes and buildings of cheap and flimsy materials, we have stripped the land of trees to hold back the mud, and have separated ourselves by race, economics, and even gender.

These types of disasters of epic proportions illustrate vividly that we are really only a moment's step from oblivion. I know that it sounds nihilistic and bleak, and that is not my intention. For most of us in the developed world, especially western nations, we try to protect ourselves from the wrath of nature. We build to code, we chart fault lines, we buy flood insurance, waterproof our homes, and take many other steps to shield ourselves from the tragedy and disaster that our sister countries around the world experience annually. We are fortunate to have been born or to live in a world with these opportunities. What the Earthquake in Haiti illustrates is that we are all connected, even if not by geography, but by the human spirit of joy and now extreme suffering.

For most of us, we will never know what it is to feel as if the world has disappeared—to not be able to find loved ones, to find shelter or food, to not have medical care for those who are injured, or to bury those who have died. What has happened on this poor island called Haiti is the next chapter in a history marked by violence, abuse, slavery, rape, illiteracy, starvation, and fear—not by just one country but many—many that are the leaders of the free world today.

Perhaps to rewrite this chapter, the world can unify to send aid, to send troops who will come to protect and not kill, and to send money to rebuild. In the biblical sense could this be the next Great Flood, which wiped out the misery of the past in order to build anew? Instead of animals on that ark, each one of us can play a part by contributing money and resources to a country—to a people—who have mainly known terror. It can start with each one of us providing that human connection to care.

When It Rains, It Pours!

Have you ever woken up and felt a pang in the pit of your stomach, knowing that it's going to be a tough day? A couple of weeks ago, I had that feeling one morning and, not surprisingly, it foreshadowed what was ahead. I woke up knowing it was the one-year anniversary of my mom's funeral so my expectation for the day was to just get through it.

I smiled for a brief moment when I noticed that it was gently raining outside, remembering how it briefly rained during the chapel service as if the heavens were crying with us. However, when I looked out my living room window, I saw the aftermath signs of a torrential downpour: broken tree limbs and mulch dispersed all over the lawn. In the past before I got my sump pumps, my basement would flood. But now I had two pumps installed and felt somewhat protected. Yet, I needed to do the check to make sure that all was okay.

My heart dropped the moment I touched the new carpet in the basement den and saw the wet imprints of my feet. Quickly, I looked into all the rooms and was greeted by wet floors and soggy rugs and carpet. Both sump pumps had failed and had actually acted as swimming pools. There was barely a single dry spot left to move anything to safe ground.

I moved fast, but knew that it was going to be a lost cause—now it was just a salvage operation. The rain kept coming and my pumps were silent. I ran to my office to use my laptop computer to search for a plumber who could fix them. But as the black cloud that centered on my home would have it, as soon as I opened my new computer the plastic connection between the screen and keyboard cracked into two. I was too numb at this point to even cry or laugh. So I did what we used to do, I used the old fashioned phone book to find help, which came in the form of a plumber who was from the Cameroon. With the use of a credit card, new pumps and cleaned out pipes, the problem was hopefully solved. Now came the ten hours of fun trying to sop up water from a carpet and pad that held it like a sponge.

Stress! We all have it, but some days are worse than others. The interesting thing was that even though this experience was exhausting and anxiety provoking, it did not come close to what I felt the year before. Losing a loved one is beyond description—the hollowness in our hearts and the pain in our souls sear throughout our beings. Nothing can soothe it but the gift of time. Perhaps, the universe was being kind to me because on August 18 I was so preoccupied to get my home, my source of security back to being whole, that my mind did not totally focus on my loss. In some ways, the physical exhaustion that came with the day was a salve to heal my wounds. In a strange way, I am grateful. Of course I'll be grateful too when the swamp aroma enveloping my home is a distant memory.

It's Only Skin Deep

Did anyone ever tell you that beauty is skin deep? I never quite understood that expression. But I did know that going for a facial was a relaxing treat that you could give yourself (or others), and that perhaps it helped to restore your vitality and healthy appearance. So after a pretty busy few weeks of travel, work and personal obligations, I decided to have a facial.

When I arrived at the spa, I was told that a new aesthetician was in training and that she wanted to try a new type of facial on me. Since I always believe that we should mentor and train others, I was more than happy to be a practice client (or shall I say 'guinea pig'). Plus, I wanted to try something new and different!

I was taken out of the cozy room with the nice soothing music and brought into what looked like an operating room with a bed underneath a bright light. I knew immediately this was not going to be typical facial, and I was more than a little curious what would happen next. It seemed I was going to experience a facial that belonged in one of my biochemistry labs. I never knew that there existed goo containing vitamins, anti-oxidants, bio-peptides (which apparently increases elastin and collagen), and even colostrum (Yes, it is breast milk from a cow and it contains growth factors and anti-inflammatory agents). It was all mixed in with algae and brushed on to my face including my eyelids and mouth.

I now was encased in a mask that resembled something from a sci-fi movie. I dared not speak or blink. Soon, this mask hardened into a rubbery like substance and was pulled off my face. I couldn't believe that my eyelashes did not come with it; I actually checked the back of my facial imprint to make sure those precious lashes were not attached to it.

I had to laugh when I was asked what products I used. For someone who first started her skin care regimen using lemon juice as an astringent because she did not have any money for the fancy stuff, I was pretty proud that I had actually graduated to drugstore specials. I do admit that I have always used good sunscreens on my skin, but that was about it. I know that staying out of the sun, drinking lots of water, not smoking, a healthy diet of fruits and vegetables, sleep and, of course, good genes were the keys to healthy looking skin. But now I know that there are more tools out there to utilize, and some include using ingredients that only a biochemist would love. There are even devices that use electrical currents or sound waves to get greater penetration of molecules through the skin. Who knew?

Of course, as I was leaving, I ended up buying a lotion and a roller that contains micro-needles to penetrate down deeper. I figured I would do my own science experiment to see if there is enhanced clarity. Could I actually reverse the years of sunbathing with baby oil while sitting in a snow bank in Colorado? Now, if I can only get 8 hours of sleep and 8 glasses of water...time will tell!

To the Center of the Earth

The world was transfixed to a remote location in the middle of Atacama Desert in Chile on October 13, 2010. Every 20 to 40 minutes, we witnessed the rebirth of 33 miners arising from the depths of the Earth in the Phoenix to the loving arms of their family members and countrymen. For over two months these men were trapped more than 2,000 feet beneath the surface of the driest location on the planet, where in some places there has never been a drop of rain on record. The irony to that is nothing rots out there, but it is just preserved as an artifact. Astronomers gather here to look into the cosmos through the pure clean sky. All of these elements came together to create one of the greatest survival stories in history.

After a mine collapsed, the miners found themselves trapped with barely any food or water. For 17 days, no one knew if they were even alive. When a small burr hole was punch through their prison cave, a note was sent back up to civilization that they were alive against unbeatable odds — rationing a spoonful of tuna or milk every other day and surviving on their sheer guts and will to see those they loved again. We have all heard similar stories in the past, but this time we could witness it moment by moment, day by day, month by month. We got to know their backgrounds, their families, and their dismal chances to be rescued.

Within days of the message, NASA sent to Chile a team of doctors to provide guidance and counsel on how to keep people alive and "well" under very remote and extreme conditions. NASA has a superb history of doing that each day as our astronauts circle the Earth every 90 minutes. Perhaps, we have become immune to that brilliant success and take it for granted, but every bodily function is assessed and every drop of food and water are precious commodities in an outpost hundreds of miles above our protective atmosphere. Everyone seemed surprised that the miners looked and seemed so vigorous when they came to the surface. For those of us who work at NASA, we know it was because of the expertise of the medical community that made that happen. It was the sacred patient-doctor relationship at its best.

The Phoenix, the life vessel that delivered the miners and their rescuers home, was a testament to creative engineering, again both within NASA and the Chilean government. As we saw with Apollo 13 after the explosion that crippled the mother ship, human ingenuity is immeasurable. The Chileans did an outstanding job working with the world community and the world community responded.

"Community" is a word that we banter about sometimes flippantly. But it is the community that can keep our spirits high, our dreams alive and our will to survive. Every man down in that cave was each other's brother; they seemed to care for one another, perhaps even fight at times, but they kept each other alive. I was not surprised to hear one miner comment that there was a 34th miner among them: their God or higher being. I always believed that the faith and love that surround a person determines how he or she will do when faced with a crisis. I have seen it with patients, our troops and even my own family members. We are all connected to each other on this planet, all made of stardust, and it is that connection that makes our universe brighter.

The Invisible Injuries of War

Editor's Note: The following is a letter to the editor — authored by Dr. Saralyn Mark and printed in the *Washington Post*.

The Oct. 3 front-page article on traumatic brain injuries, "**It changes who we are,**" tragically hit home for me.

The military is finally acknowledging that exposure to constant explosions from guns and other weapons damages the sensitive brain tissue that gives our loved ones the ability to think, remember and feel. Our family members may be returning home from the battlefield, but their invisible injuries continually destroy their spirits.

Imagine looking into the eyes of your loved one and being met by an abyss where there was once loving recognition. The pain that we feel cannot be measured by words or soothed by empty promises. Our nation needs a call to action to ensure that everyone who has served our country gets the competent care that he or she deserves.

We must ensure that our brave warriors can defend our nation and can come back and be productive members of our society and our families. If we do not, the casualties from these wars will not be reflected just by those who have died, but by families that have been destroyed

Remembering the Invisible Heroes

On Veteran's Day, we fly our flags and we attend rallies, concerts and parades to honor our military veterans. All are wonderful expressions of support and appreciation. But for some of our citizens, the war's impact goes far beyond what can be provided by these gestures.

There has been much written about the injuries of these wars on our troops—the tragic consequences of traumatic brain injuries, post traumatic stress disorders and amputations. We see these horrific wounds from every war, but this time only 1% of the American population is faced with these challenges. There is no draft or conscription; those who serve do it voluntarily and willingly. We honor their sacrifices. But there is another group that also shoulders the burden—the military family, often invisible and taken for granted.

At one time, especially after World War II, almost every family in America had a loved one who had served in the military. It was a badge of honor. That is not the case today. Even though the war in Afghanistan has gone on for almost ten years and the fighting in Iraq has topped over seven years, most families in this nation have been protected from the ravages of these wars. War is not a universally shared experience.

I recall trying to talk to some friends about what it was like to have a loved one in the military and was met with blank stares or a request to change the topic. It was not something that they wanted to hear about, as it did not impact their lives. I don't think these reactions were done out of meanness or selfishness, but war is ugly and is not an easy topic to digest. We love our freedoms and our ability to enjoy the fruits of our labor, but for some, they would rather not have to think about what it took for us to get there.

We all have to deal with stresses from our daily chores of living, but now add fear and loneliness that is only occasionally lessened by a call or message from a loved one who is deployed. These are not just long distance relationships that funny movies or comedies are built around. These are relationships that hinge on the very word or expression that can be shared across miles. It would be comforting to know that one is not alone in this experience. And that is why I hope for this Veteran's Day that we also reach out with our full hearts to families that have proudly sacrificed so much.

Blue Star Families is a non-partisan organization dedicated to improving the lives of military families through outreach, programming, and education. In 2010, they conducted a lifestyle survey to assess the needs and concerns of military families. In addition to employment difficulties for spouses and educational gaps for children (who often move from location to location), it's the anxiety over the impact of deployments of parents on children that tops the list of challenges facing modern day military families. Ninety-two percent of the responders said that the public does not understand the sacrifices that are made by military families; 79% said that they would like more support from the community for military children dealing with deployment.

As a nation, we need to care for our military families everyday, not just on special holidays. Simple acts of respect and kindness can go a long way. Volunteer in your community to help a family. It can be with basic chores or just lending a friendly ear to hear their stories over a cup of coffee. Not every military family lives on a military base and isolation can be a big issue. Invite them to be a part of your celebrations and events. Most importantly, voice your support and appreciation for what they are enduring everyday, which allows all of us to enjoy the gifts of being an American.

Roller Coasters and Cotton Candy

When I was a little girl, we use to go to Elitch Gardens Amusement Park in Denver. I loved it! The thrill of the rides and the joy of the sweet cotton candy that turned your lips fluorescent blue or pink filled me with delight. Although some of the rides made me completely nauseous, I would never think of not going back for more.

The excitement of the wooden roller coaster or rides that simulated space flight or elevator drops stirred my imagination to reach for the stars. I felt fearless, especially when my 4-foot frame was finally big enough to be strapped into those flying machines that looped upside down and all around. After fearing death, the reward was to land back on my feet and go for more cotton candy. It is funny how we all probably remember childhood memories of those warm summer nights. It was just pure exhilaration.

Little did I know that it might become a metaphor for how life would turn out. One roller coaster ride after another, one moment of fear followed by sheer excitement and happiness, pinnacles and drop-offs, speed and stagnation all in one ride. I knew that 2010 would be like that—I could sense it as it was approaching. But I strapped myself into the seat and went for the ride. I was not disappointed. I knew that there were going to be challenges—some even unexpected—but like that cotton candy at the end of the ride, there were friends, family, colleagues and neighbors waiting to help sweeten the moments.

I got through the agony of holidays and events without my beautiful mom and the loss of another precious loved one with grace and dignity to ease the void. Yet, there were high adventures in lands far away, mountains to be climbed and sunsets to be treasured. I occasionally let the heat of the sun's rays warm my shoulders and fuel my soul to keep on moving. I am ready for the next ride, but first I'm going to finish my giant ball of cotton candy!

Arizona Shooting: The Enemy Within

I left work last Friday feeling sad that our country seemed so divided to the point where there was no room for constructive dialog. As I rode the D.C. metro home, I kept thinking about a conversation I had with some friends that day. It was just 48 hours after the new Congress was sworn in and 18 hours before the Arizona massacre. I was concerned that collegiality and respect would be gone forever or at least for a very long time. Some of my friends had very different political views from me, but in the past, we could usually see eye-to-eye on some issues. But on that day, with the aroma of new power percolating through the nation's capitol, there was no room for that. The focus was on how to erode all the accomplishments that were made over the last two years while cementing a foundation for new presidential candidates and exhorting the wise decisions of the prior administration. It left me feeling a bit hopeless that we would ever be again the "United" States of America.

Some of the health programs that I had worked on for years were now being erased, even though they could serve the public well and with very little of our tax payer resources, but they had been sponsored by a Senator who was no longer there. When my neighbor called me that night, I told her that I was so worried that the polarization and anger would lead to something heinous. What I was seeing was not American politics in all its jest and candor but vitriol and hatred.

It was during a bar mitzvah luncheon that I got a message that there had been a shooting in Arizona and that a congresswoman had been shot. We all assumed that someone from the far right or from the "Tea Party" was responsible. It just seemed to be the natural course of events from the nasty fall campaign to the rhetoric exuding from the walls of Congress and blogs in cyberspace. When I learned that it was Congresswoman Giffords, whom I met during aerospace briefings on Capitol Hill and the wife of a fellow NASA employee-astronaut Mark Kelly and a member of the Tucson congregation that I had joined in 2004, I was devastated. Then to learn about all the other victims that were slaughtered outside a grocery store filled me with a sense of despair that I had not felt in a very long time.

The reaction following this event reminds me of what we saw after other tragedies. While some had more casualties, this one struck a slightly different chord. I think it's because of two reasons. First, a beloved congresswoman and the wife of a space hero was nearly assassinated which has not happened in our recent history. She also represented one of the most sacred institutions in this country: a government 'of,' 'by' and 'for the people.' By attacking her, we were all attacked. Secondly, because we all thought that it was caused by someone with political rancor to silence the opposition, we finally realized how far the pendulum had swung—from a civilized society to one steeped in vengeance and retribution. These were atrocities that happened in other countries, not ours.

As the information unfolded, it became clear that the perpetrator was a severely disturbed man who had access to guns and lots of ammunition. This generated more discussion about the inadequacies of our mental health system and the ease to acquire guns that have no reason to be used in our society, not even for hunting animals. A friend from overseas commented that Americans need to realize that the British redcoats have left these shores and Native Americans are no longer attacking or trying to defend their territory. So who is now the enemy? I am reminded of a saying "We have seen the enemy and he is us." With all our military and money fighting Al Qaida and the Taliban, the terrorists that have created some of the most recent horror have been home grown: Oklahoma City, Virginia Tech, Columbine, and Fort Hood to name but a few.

Of course, discussions ensued that this was the outgrowth of the divisive language and venom that spewed from the lips of politicians and commentators and regular Americans following along that fostered an environment that even a deranged man would be affected—not being able to differentiate fact from fiction. I do believe that it is possible, but I also feel something more ethereal. I have often said that we are all connected to each other on this planet. That which impacts one can impact all of us. We are linked together from the beginning of time. We cannot survive if we do not come together to care for one another, to heal one another, to protect one another. At the end of the day, what is important is the kindness that we have shared and the love that we have given. Nothing else matters.

Delivery in the Dirt

Imagine delivering your baby in the dirt, in the mud, stark naked, with no one to help you. Imagine having to pull out the hair on your head to use it to tie off the umbilical cord. Now imagine scrounging around in the dark for a piece of wood to sever the umbilical cord from the placenta. These are not images from a horror movie—it is the cruel reality of life in the death camps in the Congo.

On March 3, I spoke at the United Nations for an event for the Commission on the Status of Women. I served on a panel along with reps from France, the UK and Switzerland. We were asked to present how medical innovation and education can transform the lives of women around the world. Science, Technology, Engineering and Mathematics (STEM) were the buzzwords of the session. Everyone discussed how we needed to educate girls to go into these fields in order to secure the next generation of innovators and leaders. After I presented data from the new White House Report on the Status of Women (first report in almost 50 years), STEM programs sponsored by NASA and the private sector and how sex and gender influences medical technology, I took questions from the standing room only audience. That is when I heard from Rose.

Rose was from the Congo. After her husband was murdered by a band of rebels, she and her eight children were taken to death camps far from her home. There she was raped and tortured. When she learned that she was pregnant, she had no one to help her. So on a dark night in the mud, she delivered her baby by herself. Eventually another woman took off her own clothing to give her something to wear. Somehow Rose survived this horrific ordeal and promised herself and her children that she would not be silent and alone anymore.

Miraculously, she survived these camps and made it to the U.S. Rose now works as an advocate and activist to raise awareness of what women endure around the world. As our panel focused on higher education, her goal was to help girls learn how to read and write-to spell their names, to be able to get a job.

It has been shown that when a girl is educated and can work, she gives 90% of what she makes back to her family, back to her community which can stabilize her country.

I can summarize my talk in just 6 words—"Educate a girl, save a Nation"

Up in the Air

"Is there a doctor on board?" Those are six words that can get
every doctor's heart beating a bit faster at 36,000 feet above the
ground. I have heard them several times while flying, but the most
recent event, which happened a week ago, changed the course for not
only my plane trip but also for my holiday in Ireland. I was
finally taking a vacation to celebrate my birthday and get some
relaxation; or so I thought. Just as I was settling in to watch a fun
movie, the screen paused for the announcement asking for a doctor. I
pushed my call button, and immediately, a flight attendant appeared
at my side. In some ways, I felt like I had entered the ER and was asking
a nurse about the new patients. Funny how memories kick in with
certain triggers.   The flight attendant told me that two children were
quite ill and their mother was very concerned. I told her that I was not
a pediatrician (in fact I am a geriatrician-the opposite end of the
spectrum), but I would do my best. So in my stocking feet, I walked
down the aisle to assess the situation. We were only an hour into the
flight so if it was necessary we could divert and turn back to the U.S.
A woman was sitting next to two ill appearing children who
kept reaching for their vomit bags. They were twins around the age of
nine and were flying home from New Orleans to Ireland. Apparently,
one of their family members in New Orleans had previously been ill
with GI symptoms so this could have been contagious.   It is hard to
examine or get a history when you are standing in an aisle surrounded
by passengers on all sides. I was also concerned that the kids could be
quite dehydrated and needed to lie down and if they were infectious,
it was better to isolate them a bit from the other passengers. I learned
that there were a few empty seats in first class and asked for them to
be moved. Once we got them up to the front of the plane, I was able
to check them and learn more about them. It is also interesting how
one learns to practice medicine in 'extreme environments' when you
have to do that. NASA where I work is known for the most extreme
environments and I knew that we could do fine at 36,000 feet if we
could do fine 400 miles about the Earth's atmosphere. Although the
family was moved, the doctor was not allowed to stay in first class so
every few minutes the flight attendant would come back and ask me
questions and I would get to walk up the aisle to see my new patients.

At one point, I vetoed the advice from ground medical support since I was with my little patients and could see how they were doing—the so-called 'eye ball test.' Over the next few hours, we dealt with nausea, vomiting, fever, body aches and dizziness. I found creative approaches to take care of all these signs and symptoms. As the plane was landing and wheel chairs were waiting for my young patients to take them to a medical facility, their mother and I exchanged information. It turned out they owned a castle in a beautiful part of Ireland.

The next day, I received an email from their mom thanking me for helping her through the night and offering for me to come and visit. I decided to come and see them on the Dingle peninsula the following weekend since I heard it was a very beautiful part of the country and I could celebrate my birthday with some new friends. So on that day, surrounded by people who were strangers at 36,000 feet, but now my new friends in their home, I blew out the candles on my birthday pie. The best gift was to see the children run, play and laugh. There is no better present for a doctor who just happened to answer the call "Is there a doctor on board?"

Peace of Mind

I saw the Dalai Lama a few months ago up close and personal with 10,000 of my friends on the lawn of the Capitol. On a very hot summer morning under a bright blue sky with the iconic landmarks of Washington, DC in the background, the Dalai Lama had an intimate conversation with all of us. A jovial, funny and warm-hearted soul, he shared his wisdom and insights on world peace and the search for inner happiness.

Not far from the stage, I sat down on a plastic sheet on the lawn offered to me by a woman in formal dress from her native land of Bhutan. Her family had been killed when she was a child in Tibet. From Bhutan, she made it to India and then on to San Francisco and was now a nurse in a intensive care unit at Stanford. She generously shared her sunscreen and her knowledge of Buddhism, the Tibetan language and costumes. As I was melting into the plastic, I was mesmerized by the diverse and respectful audience. People stood when they should, clapped when it was appropriate, shared their water and their books on traditional prayers. I felt quite safe and transfixed as if I had entered a new land, a new culture far from my home which was only 10 miles away.

We all eagerly awaited the arrival of the Dalai Lama-the spiritual leader of Tibet who recently resigned as the political leader saying it was hypocritical thinking that one could do both. The event was moderated by Whoopie Goldberg who did a lovely job of using humor and sincerity—you could tell that she was in awe of her new position.

When the Dalai Lama came onto the stage, we all rose and then very quietly sat down to listen to this wise man with a delightful smile and an easy-going manner. He said that he did not prepare any remarks-in fact, he never liked to prepare remarks and then he embarked on a brilliant one-hour discourse on how and why it is important to achieve inner peace. Love, compassion, trust, warm-heartedness are the hallmarks of a healthy mind and life.

When one faces adversity and people who make life difficult, accept that these are opportunities to practice patience and tolerance. I know that this is a tough lesson to accept, but it does make sense and changes one's outlook on life. He said that no one is immune from troubles, but all of us are destined for happiness. The two major events in life are birth and death and the rest we do with people. We are social beings-each one of us can change the world and by doing that, peace can be achieved. Inner beauty is what is important, the rest is window dressing (my words) and fleeting.

My new book 'Stellar Medicine: A Journey Through the Universe of Women's Health' (Brick Tower Press) will be released this month. One of my chapters, "The Stardust Connection" which discusses faith, spirituality and healing, is one of my favorite chapters for book readings. The messages in this chapter, namely, that we are all connected from the beginning of time since we are stardust and that spirituality is as important to health as the physical elements that we can measure. I have shared that chapter with the senior echelon of medicine, military and government women, and the general public and have seen that these messages resonate with all audiences.

What I found so inspiring is that I came to my beliefs out my own experiences not from reading or studying others' works. So when I heard the Dalai Lama share the same insights that I do in my book, I was joyous. He calls it "secular spirituality"—a belief that is not based in religion or faith, but on our divine right and ability to find inner happiness, a calm mind, and a generous spirit to connect with others. Through this, our health can improve and wellness can be achieved. He mentioned that he spoke to scientists who confirmed that blood pressure can decrease and even recovery from surgery can be influenced. I believe in this wholeheartedly.

There are moments in life that are transformative and this was one of them for me. Peace of mind-so simple, so divine!

SOURCES

Chapter One: A Pandemic of Misinformation

Bishop, E. Myth or fact: Feed a cold, Starve a fever. *DukeHealth.org*. March 3, 2008.

Burns, A. van der Mensbrugghe, D. Timmer, H. Evaluating the economic consequences of avian influenza: Updated study based on originally published in a slightly different form in the World Bank's. June 2006 edition of the *Global Development Finance*.

Condon, S. 10 health care reform myths. *CBSNews.com*. August 6, 2009.

Engler, RJM. et al. Half-vs-full-dose trivalent inactivated influenza vaccine (2004-2005), age, dose, and sex effects on immune responses. *Arch Intern Med*. 2008; 168(22): 2405-2414.

Gionis, TA. et al. Dead bodies, disaster, and the myths about them: is public health law misinformed? *American Journal of Disaster Medicine*. 2007 Jul-Aug; 2(4): 173-88.

http://www.cdc.gov/Flu/about/qa/misconceptions.htm

http://www.cdc.gov/H1N1flu/antiviral.htm

http://www.globalsecurity.org/security/ops/hsc-scen-3_flu-antigenic.htm

Izzedine, V. et al. Antiviral drug-Induced nephrotoxicity. *American Journal of Kidney Disease*. 2005;45(5): 804-17.

Lappe, JM. et al. Vitamin D and calcium supplementation reduces cancer risk: Results of a Randomized Trail. *American Journal of Clinical Nutrition*. 2007 June;85(6): 1586-91.

Louie, JK. et al. Factors associated with death or hospitalization due to pandemic 2009 Influenza A(H1N1) infection in California. *The Journal of the American Medical Association*. 2009; 302(17): 1896-1902.

Rubin, R. Lessons learned from the 1976 swine flu 'fiasco.' *USA Today*. May 5, 2009.

Slocum, J. Executive Director, Funeral Consumers Alliance. Dead bodies and disease: The 'danger' that doesn't exist." Funeral Ethics Organization Newsletter, Spring/Summer 2006.

Szekeres-Bartho J, et al. The immunological pregnancy protective effect of progesterone is manifested via controlling cytokine production. *Am J Reprod Immunol* 1996;35:348-51.

Van den Brink, GR. et al. Feed a cold, starve a fever. Clinical and Diagnostic Laboratory Immunology. 2002 Jan; 9(1): 182-3.

World Health Organization. Public health risk assessment and interventions: Earthquake: Haiti. Communicable Disease Working Group on Emergencies. 2010 Jan.

Chapter Two: Hair Dye and the Killer Bra

Albrektsen, G, et al. Breast cancer risk by age at birth, time since birth, and time intervals between births. *British Journal of Cancer*. 2005;92: 167-75.

American Cancer Society (ACS). 5 most common cancer myths. http://www.cancer.org/MyACS/Eastern/AreaHighlights/5-most-common-cancer-myth. Accessed Dec 2011.

Anderson JL. et al. Evaluation of C-reactive protein, an inflammatory marker, and infectious serology as risk factors for coronary artery disease and myocardial infarction. *J Am Coll Cardiol* 1998;32: 35-41.

Andriankaja, OM. et al. The use of different measurements and definitions of periodontal disease in the study of the association between periodontal disease and risk of myocardial infraction. *Journal of Periodontology*. 2006 Jun;77(6): 1067-73.

Mirick, DK. et al. Antiperspirant Use and the Risk of Breast Cancer. *Journal of the National Cancer Institute*. 2002 Oct;94(20): 1578-80.

Archer, J. et al. Dioxin and furan levels found in tampons. *Journal of Women's Health.* 2005 May;14(4): 311-315.

Brind, J. et al. Induced abortion as an independent risk factor for breast cancer; a comprehensive review and meta-analysis. *Journal of Epidemiology and Community Health* 1996;59: 481-96.

Cook, LS. et al. Hair product use and the risk of breast cancer in young women. *Cancer Causes and Controls.* 1999;10(6): 551-9.

Gallup, G. et al. Does semen have antidepressant properties? *Archives of Sexual Behavior.* 2002; 31(3) :289-93.

Gazzaley, A. et al. Top-down suppression deficit underlies working memory impairment in normal aging. *Nature Neuroscience.* 2005 Oct;8(10): 1298-300.

Jones, J. Can rumors cause cancer? *The Journal of the National Cancer Institute.* 2000; 92:1469-71.

Katz, Joel T. et al. "Bacteria and Coronary Atheroma, More Fingerprints but No Smoking Gun" Circulation." 113:920-922. 2006.

Kramer, S.M. Fact or fiction? Underwire bras cause cancer. *Scientific America.* April 19, 2007

Martineau, LC. et al. Anti-diabetic properties of the Canadian lowbush blueberry Vaccinium angustifolium Ait. *Phytomedicine.* 2006 Nov;13(9-10): 612-23.

Mutti, DO. et al. Parental myopia, near work, school achievement, and children refractive error. *Investigative Ophthalmology and Visual Science.* 2002 Dec;43(12) :3633-40.

Ott, SJ. et al. Detection of diverse bacterial signatures in atherosclerotic lesions of patients with coronary heart disease. *Circulation.* 2006;113: 929—937

Rennard, BO. et al. Chicken soup inhibits neutrophil chemotaxis in vitro 2000. *Chest.* 2009 Nov;136(5 Suppl): e29.

Scialli, AR. Tampons, dioxins, and endometriosis. *Reproductive Toxicology.* 2001 May;15(3): 231-8.

Tanielian, T. and Jaycox, LH, eds., "Invisible Wounds of War: Psychological and Cognitive Injuries, Their Consequences, and Services to Assist Recovery, Santa Monica, Calif.": RAND Corporation, MG-720-CCF, 2008, 492 pp.

Weaver, K. Interaction between broad-spectrum antibiotics and the combined oral contraceptive pill. A literature review." *Contraception.* 1999 Feb;59(2): 71-8.

Wizemann T.M., Pardue M, eds. "Exploring the Biological Contributions to Human Health: Does Sex Matter?" Committee on Understanding the Biology of Sex and Gender Differences. Washington, D.C.: National Academy of Sciences, 2001. Wong, L. et al. Education, reading, and familial tendency as risk factors for myopia in Hong King fisherman. *Journal of Epidemiology and Community Health.* 1993;47:50-53.

World Health Organization, International Agency for Research on Cancer. Occupational exposure of hairdressers and barbers and personal use of hair colourants' some hair dyes, cosmetic colourants, industrial dyestuffs and aromatic amines. *IRC Monographs on the Evaluation of Carcinogenic Risks to Humans.* 1993; 57.

Chapter Three: Womb on the Moon

Carlson, K J., et al. Indications of hysterectomy. *The New England Journal of Medicine.* 1993 March;328:856-60.

Rodrigues, I. et al. Effectiveness of emergency contraceptive pills between 72 and 120 hours after unprotected sexual intercourse. *American Journal of Obstetrics & Gynecology,* 2001 March;184(4): 531-537.

Zhoa, SZ., et al. The Cost of Inpatient Endometriosis Treatment: An Analysis Based on the Healthcare Cost and Utilization Project Nationwide Inpatient Sample. *American Journal of Managed Care.* 1998 August;4(8): 1127-34.

Chapter Four: Global Warming and More Hot Flashes

Albertazzi P. et al. The effect of dietary soy supplementation on hot flushes. *Obstet Gynecol.* 1998;91:6-11.

Anderson GL. et al. Effects of conjugated equine estrogen in postmenopausal women with hysterectomy: the Women's Health Initiative randomized controlled trial. JAMA. 2004 Apr 14;291(14): 170-12.

Barton D. et al. Prospective evaluation of vitamin E for hot flashes in breast cancer survivors. *Journal of Clinical Oncology*. 1998;16:495-500.

Becker, E. et al. Is black cohosh a safe and effective substitute for hormone replacement therapy? *Journal of the American Academy of Physician Assistants*. 2009 Sep;22(9): 54-5.

Chlebowski, RT. et al. Estrogen plus progestin and breast cancer incidence and mortality in postmenopausal women. JAMA 2010 Oct 20;304(15): 1684-92.

Davis, SR. Tran, J. Testosterone influences libido and well being in women. *Trends in Endocrinology and Metabolism*. 2001 Jan-Feb;12(1): 33-7.

Glazier MG. Bowman MA. A review of the evidence for the use of Phytoestrogens as a replacement for traditional estrogen replacement therapy. *Arch Intern Med*. 2001;161:1161-72.

Gordon N. Sobel D. Tarazona E. Use of and interest in alternative therapies among adult primary care clinicians and adult members in a large health maintenance organization. *West J Med*. 1998;169:153-161.

Hammar M. Berg G. Lindgren R. Does physical exercise influence the frequency of postmenopausal hot flushes? *Acta Obstet Gynecol Scand*. 1990;69(5): 409-12.

Henderson, VW. et al. Estrogen exposures and memory at midlife. *American Academy of Neurology*. 2003 Apr;60(8): 1369-71.

Ivarsson, T. Spetz, A.C. Hammer, M. Physical exercise and vasomotor symptoms in postmenopausal women. *Maturitas*. 1998;29:139-46.

Kang, HJ., Ansbacher, R., Hammoud, MM. Use of alternative and complementary medicine in menopause. *International Journal of Gynecology & Obstetrics*, 1990;79(3): 195-207..

Krebs, EE. et al. Phytoestrogens for treatment of menopausal symptoms: A systematic review. *Obstetrics & Gynecology*: 2004 Oct;104(4): 824-36.

Manson, JE. et al. Estrogen therapy and coronary-artery calcification. *New England Journal of Medicine*. 2007 Jun 21;356(25): 2591-602.

Seeling, MS. Interrelationship of magnesium and estrogen in cardiovascular and bone disorders, eclampsia, migraine and

premenstrual syndrome. *Journal Amer. College of Nutrition* 1993
    Aug;12(4): 442-58.
Newton, KM. et al. Use of alternative therapies for menopause
    symptoms: results of a population-based survey. *Obstetrics &
    Gynecology.* 2002 July;100(1): 18-25.
Shumaker, SA. et al. Estrogen Plus Progestin and the Incidence of
    Dementia and Mild Cognitive Impairment in Postmenopausal
    Women. *The Journal of the American Medical Association.* 2003
    May;289(20): 2651-62.
Vincent, A. et al. Acupuncture for hot flashes: a randomized, sham
    controlled clinical study. *Menopause.* 2007 Jan-Feb;14(1): 45-52.
Weber, M. Mapstone, M. Memory complaints and memory
    performance in the menopausal transition." *Menopause.* 2009
    July-Aug;16(4): 694-700.

Chapter Five: Cosmic Cosmetology
American Heart Association. Heart disease and stroke statistics: 2004
    update.
    http://americanheart.org/downloadable/heart/1072969766940HS
    Stats2004Update.pdf. Accessed January 15, 2004.
Baugh, GS. Effects of team gender and racial composition on
    perceptions of team performance in cross-functional teams.
    Group and Organization Management. 1997;22(3): 366-83.
Briton, NJ. Hall, JA. Beliefs about female and male nonverbal
    communications. *Sex Roles.* 1995 Jan;32(1-2): 79-90.
Dewing, P. et al. Direct regulation of adult brain function by the
    male-specific factor SRY. *Current Biology.* 2006 Feb;16(4): 41520.
Eskes,T. Haanen, C. Why do women live longer than men? *Eur J
    Obstet Gynecol Reprod Biol.* 2007 Aug;133(2): 126-133.
Fairweather, D. Frisancho-Kiss, S. Rose, NR. Sex differences in
    autoimmune disease from a pathological perspective. *American
    Journal of Pathology.* 2008 Sep;173(3): 600-9.
Friedman, B. et al. The watcher and the watched: social judgments
    about privacy in a public place. *Human-Computer Interaction.*
    2006 May;21(2): 235-72.
Gale, EA. Gillespie, KM. Diabetes and gender. *Diabetologia* 2001
    Jan;44(1): 3-15.

Harm, DL. et al. Invited review: gender issues related to spaceflight: a NASA perspective. *Journal of Applied Physiology*. 2001 Nov;91(5): 2374-83.

Hay, AM. Bladder cancer: inequalities in bladder cancer survival. *Nature Reviews Urology* 2009 April;6: 177.

Hollowell JG. et al. Serum. TSH, T(4), and thyroid antibodies in the United States population (1988 to 1994): National Health and Nutrition Examination Survey (NHANES III). *J Clin Endocrinol Metab*. 2002;87:489-99.

Larsen P.R., Davies T.F., Hay I.D., The thyroid gland. Wilson JD, Foster DW, Kronenberg HM, Larsen PR, eds. *Williams Textbook of Endocrinology*. 9th ed. Philadelphia, PA: WB Saunders, 1998: 389-515.

MacGeorge, EL. et al. The myth of gender cultures: similarities outweigh differences in men's and women's provision of and responses to supportive communication. *Sex Roles*. 2004 Feb;50(3-4): 143-75.

Mungan NA. et al. Gender differences in stage-adjusted bladder cancer survival. *Urology*. 2000 Jun;55(6):876-80.

Neumayer, E. et al. The gendered nature of natural disasters: the impact of catastrophic events on the gender gap in life expectancy, 1981-2002." *Annals of the Association of American Geographers*. 2007 Sep;97(3): 551-566.

Nicholson WK. et al. Prevalence of postpartum thyroid dysfunction: a quantitative review. *Thyroid*. 2006;16: 573-582.

Pietschmann P. et al. Osteoporosis: an age-related and gender-specific disease—a mini review. *Gerontology*. 2008; 55:3-12.

Qaseem A. et al. Screening for osteoporosis in men: a clinical practice guideline from the American College of Physicians. *Ann Intern Med*. 2008 May 6;148(9): 680-84.

Ridker, PM. A randomized trial of low-dose aspirin in the primary prevention of cardiovascular disease in women. *The New England Journal of Medicine*. 2005 March;352: 1293-304.

Royce, RA. et al. Gender differences in survival after AIDS diagnosis: U.S. surveillance data. International Conference on AIDS. 1991 Jun 16-21; 7: 331.

Tremblay, L et al. Gender differences in perception of self-orientation: software or hardware? *Perception* 2004;33(3): 329-37.

University Of California, Irvine (2005, January 22). Intelligence in men and women is a gray and white matter. *ScienceDaily*. Retrieved September 12, 2009.

Van Den Eeden, SK. et al. Incidence of Parkinson's disease: variation by age, gender, and race/ethnicity. *American Journal of Epidemiology*. 2003 Jun;157(11): 1015-22.

Vogel, SA. Gender differences in intelligence, language, visual-motor abilities and academic achievement in students with learning disabilities. *Journal of Learning Disabilities*. 1990;23(1): 44-52.

Wizemann TM, Pardue M. eds. Exploring the biological contributions to human health: does sex matter?" Committee on Understanding the Biology of Sex and Gender Differences. Washington, DC: National Academy of Sciences, 2001.

Zang, EA. Wynder, EL. Differences in lung cancer risk between men and women: examination of the evidence. *Journal of the National Cancer Institute*. 1996 Feb;88(3-4): 183-92.

Chapter Six: A Nation of Ghosts

Alvarez, L. Female soldiers balance devotions: country, children. *The New York Times*. September 30, 2009.

Benedict, H. For women warriors, deep wounds, little care. *New York Times*. May 26, 2008.

Chandola, T. et al. Chronic stress at work and the metabolic syndrome: prospective study. *BMJ* 2006 March;332: 521-25.

Davis, T. Wood, P. Substance abuse and sexual trauma in a female veteran population. *Journal of Substance Abuse Treatment*. 1999:16(2): 123-127.

Federman, D. et al. Patient Gender Affects Skin Cancer Screening Practices and Attitudes Among Veterans. *Southern Medical Journal*. 2008 May;101(5): 513-518.

Friedman, MJ. Prevention of psychiatric problems among limitary personnel and their spouses. *The New England Journal of Medicine*. 2010 Jan 14;362(2): 168-70.

Gibbs, D. et al. Child maltreatment in enlisted soldiers' families during combat-related deployments. *Journal of the American Medical Association*. 2007 Aug;298(5): 528-535.

Hill, JJ. et al. Separating deployment-related traumatic brain injury and posttraumatic stress disorder in veterans: preliminary findings from the Veterans Affairs traumatic brain injury screening program. *Am J Phys Med Rehabil*. 2009 Dec; 88(12): 1043-4.

Holbrook, TL. et al. Morphine use after combat injury in Iraq and post-traumatic stress disorder. *The New England Journal of Medicine*. 2010 Jan;362(2): 110-117.

http://www.boston.com/news/nation/washington/articles/2009/07/06/more_female_veterans_are_winding_up_homeless/

http://www.raconline.org/info_guides/veterans/veteransfaq.php#center

http://www.usnews.com/news/national/articles/2009/07/31/female-veterans-fight-for-healthcare.html

http://www.worldatlases.com/gi/cltr_MS.pdf

Huebner, AJ. Parental deployment and youth in military families, exploring uncertainty and ambiguous loss. *Family Relations*. 2007 Apr;56: 112-122.

Jensen, PS. et al. Prevalence of mental disorder in military children and adolescents: findings form a two-stage community survey. *Journal of the American Academy of Child & Adolescent Psychiatry*. 1995 Nov;34(11): 151-24.

Jervis, R. Despite rule, U.S. women on front line in Iraq war. *USA Today*. June 26, 2005.

King, D. et al. Posttraumatic stress disorder in a national sample of female and male Vietnam veterans: Risk factors, war-zone stressors, and resilience-recovery variables. *Journal of Abnormal Psychology*. 1999 Feb;108(1): 164-70.

Mansfield, A. et al. Deployment and the use of mental health services among U.S. army wives. *The New England Journal of Medicine*. 2010 Jan;362(2): 101-9.

McKelvey, T. Life as an American female soldier. *Marie Claire*. 2007.

Okie, S. Traumatic Brain Injury in the War Zone. *The New England Journal of Medicine*. 2005 May 19;352(20): 2043-2047.

Schiraldi, Glenn R. "The Post-Traumatic Stress Disorder
    Sourcebook." McGraw, New York, 2009.
Strowbridge, NF. "Musculoskeletal injuries in female soldiers: analysis
    of cause and type of injury. J R Army Med Corps. 2002
    Sep;148(3): 256-8.
Tanielian, T. Jaycox, LH. eds. Invisible Wounds of War: Psychological
    and Cognitive Injuries, Their Consequences, and Services to
    Assist Recovery, Santa Monica, Calif." RAND Corporation,
    MG-720-CCF, 2008, 492 pp.
United States Department of Defense. "Report of the Defense Task
    Force on Sexual Assault in the Military Services." December
    2009.
United States Government Accountability Office, VA Healthcare.
    Mild traumatic brain injury screening and evaluation
    implemented for OEF/OIF Veterans, but challenges remain. ,
    GAO-08-276. February 2008.
United States Government Accountability Office, Homeless Veterans
    Programs. Improved communications and follow-up could
    enhance the grant and per diem program. GAO-06-859. Sept
    2006.
United States Government Accountability Office. VA Healthcare.
    Preliminary findings on VA's provision of healthcare services to
    women veterans. GAO-09-899T. July 2009.
Yaeger, D. et al. DSM-IV diagnosed posttraumatic stress disorder in
    women veterans with and without military sexual trauma. *Journal
    of General Internal Medicine*. 2006 March;21(3): S65-S69.
Zoroya, G. Troops' kids feel war toll. *USA Today*. June 6, 2009.

Chapter Seven: Sex, Chocolate, Wine, and Shopping
Bancroft, J. Vukadinovic, Z. Sexual addiction, sexual compulsivity,
    sexual impulsivity, or what? Toward a theoretical model. *The
    Journal of Sex Research*. 2004 Aug;41(3): 225-34.
Black, D. A review of compulsive buying disorder. *World Psychology*.
    2007 Feb;6(1): 14-8.
Brody, S. Tillmann, HC. The post-orgasmic prolactin increase
    following intercourse is greater than following masturbation and

suggests greater satiety. *Biological Psychology*. 2006 March;71(3): 312-5.

Brody, S. Blood pressure reactivity to stress is better for people who recently had penile-vaginal intercourse than for people who had other or no sexual activity. *Biological Psychology*. 2006 Feb;71(2): 214-22.

Brown, L. et al. The biological responses to resveratrol and other polyphenols from alcoholic beverages. *Alcoholism Clinical and Experimental Research*. 2009 Sep;33(9): 1513-23.

Bruinsma, K. & Taren, DL. Chocolate food or drug? *Journal of the American Dietetic Association*. 1999;99(10): 1249-56.

Charnetski, C. Brennan, F. Sexual frequency and salivary immunoglobulin A. *Psychological Reports*. 2004;94: 839-44. 2004.

Chen, WY. et al. Moderate alcohol consumption during adult life, drinking patterns, and breast cancer risk. JAMA. 2011;306(17): 1884-90.

Davey Smith, G. et al. Sex and death: are they related? Findings from the Caerphilly cohort study. *BMJ*. 1997 Dec 20-27;315(7123): 1641-1644.

Ebrahim, S. et al. Sexual intercourse and risk of ischaemic stroke and coronary heart disease; the Caerphilly study. *Journal of Epidemiology and Community Health*. 2005;56: 99-102.

Gallup, G. et al. "Does semen have antiDepressant properties?" *Archives of Sexual Behavior*. 2002;31: 289-293.

http://www.mayoclinic.com/health/red-wine/HB00089

Jerlhag, E. et al. Requirement of central ghrelin signaling for alcohol reward. Proceedings of the National Academy of Sciences. 2009 July;106(27): 11318-23.

Kosfeld, M. et al. Oxytocin increases trust in humans. *Nature*. 2005 June;435: 673-676.

Lee, HJ. et al. Oxytocin: The great facilitator of life. *Progress in Neurobiology*. 2009 June:88(2): 127-51.

Lejoyeux, M. Phenomenology and psychopathology of uncontrolled buying. *The American Journals of Psychiatry*. 1996;153: 1524-1529.

Light, K. et al. More frequent partner hugs and higher oxytocin levels are linked to lower blood pressure and heart rate in premenopausal women. *Biological Psychology*. 2005 April;69(1): 5-21.

McShea, A. et al. Clinical benefit and preservation of flavonols in dark chocolate manufacturing. *Nutrition Reviews*. 2008 Nov;66(11): 630-41.

Raymond, NC. et al. Treatment of compulsive sexual behavior with Naltrexone and serotin reuptake inhibitors: two case studies. *International Clinical Psychopharmacology*. 2002 July;17(4): 201-5.

Rehm, J. et al. Alcohol drinking cessation and its effect on esophageal and head and neck cancers: A pooled analysis. *International Journal of Cancer*. 2007 May;121(5): 1132-7.

Sellers, TA., et al. Dietary folate intake, alcohol, and risk of breast cancer in a prospective study of postmenopausal women. *Epidemiology*. 2001 July;12(4): 420-8.

Serefini, M. et al. Plasma antioxidants from chocolate. *Nature*. 2003 Aug 28;424(6952): 1013.

Taubert, D. et al. Chocolate and blood pressure in elderly individuals with isolated systolic hypertension. *Journal of the American Medical Association*. 2003 Aug 27;290(8): 1029-30.

Uryvaev, Y. Petrov, G. Extremely low doses of oxytocin reduce pain sensitivity in men. *Bulletin of Experimental Biology and Medicine*. 1996 Nov;112(5): 1071-3.

Whipple, B. Komisaruk, BR. Analgesia produced in women by gential self-stimulation. *The Journal of Sex Research*. 1998;24(1): 130-40.

White, J. Labarba, R. The effects of tactile and kinesthetic stimulation on neonatal development in the premature infant. *Developmental Psychobiology*. 1976 Nov;9(6): 569-77.

Chapter Eight: The Stardust Connection

Asser SM., Swan R. Child fatalities from religion-motivated medical neglect. *Pediatrics*. 1998;101: 625-629.

Atwood, K. The ongoing problem with the National Center for Complementary and Alternative Medicine. The Committee for Skeptical Inquiry. 2003 Oct;27(5). http://www.csicop.org/si/show/ongoing_problem_with_the_natio nal_center.

Canter, P. Insufficient evidence to conclude whether or not
     Transcendental Meditation decreases blood pressure: results of a
     systematic review of randomized clinical trials. *J Hypertens.* 2004
     Nov;11: 1107-10.

Collins, FS. The Language of God. Free Press. 2006.

Fuedtner, C. et al. Spiritual care needs of hospitalized children and
     their families: a national survey of pastoral care providers'
     perceptions. *Pediatrics.* 2003 Jan;111(1): e67-e72.

Galaneter, M. Spirituality, evidence-based medicine, and Alcoholics
     Anonymous." *The American Journal of Psychiatry.* 165: 1514-
     1517, December 2008.

Gupta, S. Cheating Death: The Doctors and Medical Miracles that
     are Saving Lives Against All Odds. Wellness Central. Hatchette
     Book Group. 2009.

http://abcnews.go.com/Technology/Apollo11MoonLanding/Story?id=
     8124267&page=1

http://archives.chicagotribune.com/2009/nov/01/science/chi-tc-
     health-religion-1031-1101nov01

http://www.cancer.org/

http://health.discovery.com/centers/sleepdreams/experts/garfield.html

http://www.law.fsu.edu/library/flsupct/77067/op-77067.pdf

http://www.lifepositive.com/Body/ayurveda/ayurveda-in-india.asp

http://www.noetic.org/about.cfm

http://www.time.com/time/arts/article/0,8599,1545682,00.html

Hypericum Depression Trial Study Group. Effect of hypericum
     perforatum (St. John's wort) in major depressive disorder: a
     randomized controlled trial. *Journal of the American Medical
     Association.* 2003 Apr 10;287(14): 1500-4.

Irwin MR. et al. Effects of a behavioral intervention, tai chi chich, on
     varicella zoster-virus specific immunity and health functioning in
     older adults. *Psychosomatic Medicine.* 2003;65(5): 824-30.

King, DE. Bushwick, B. Beliefs and attitudes of hospital inpatients
     about faith healing and prayer. *The Journal of Family Practice.*
     1994 Oct;39(4): 349-352.

Krippner, Stanley C. "Conflicting perspectives on shamans and
     shamanism: Points and counterpoints." *American Psychologist.* Vol
     57(11), Nov 2002, 962-977.

Kulik, JA. Mahleer, HI. Social support and recovery from surgery. *Health Psychology.* 1989;8(2): 221-238.

Liu, J. et al. Evaluation of extracts of plant extracts for the potential treatment of menopausal symptoms. *Journal of Agricultural Chemistry.* 2001;49(5): 2472-9.

Llinas, R. Churchland, P. The mind-brain continuum: sensory process. Massachusetts Institute of Technology. 1996.

Lord, MB. Mary Baker Eddy: A Concise Story of Her Life and Work. Davis and Bond, 1918.

Luria, I. (1988a). Eytz chaim [The tree of life]. In C., Vital (Ed.), Kitvei Ari [Writings of Ari] (Vol. 1-2). Jerusalem: Vedebsky.

Morse, M. et al. Near-death experience in a pediatric population. A preliminary report. *American Journal of Disease of Children.* 1985 June;139(6): 595-600.

Paul-Labrador, M. et al. Effects of randomized controlled trial of transcendental meditation on components of the metabolic syndrome in subjects with coronary heart disease. *Archives of Internal Medicine.* 2006 Jun 12;166(11): 1218-24.

Ramachandran, V. The evolutionary biology of self-deception, laughter, dreaming and depression: some clues from anosognosia. *Medical Hypotheses.* 1996;47(5): 347-362.

Saper, RB. Heavy metal content of ayurvedic herbal medicine products. *The Journal of the American Medical Association.* 2004;292: 2868-2873.

Schneider, RH. Long-term effects of stress reduction on mortality in persons > 55 years of age with systemic hypertension. *American Journal of Cardiology.* 2005;95: 1060-4.

Simpson, SM. Near death experience: a concept analysis as applied to nursing. *Journal of Advanced Nursing.* 2001 Nov; 36(4): 520-526.

Simpson, WF. Comparative longevity in a college cohort of Christian Scientists. *The Journal of the American Medical Association.* 1989;262(12): 1657-1658.

St. John Dowling. "Lourdes cures and their medical assessment." *Journal of the Royal Society of Medicine.* 1984 Aug;77: 634-8.

Taylor, M. Imaginary Companions and the Children Who Create Them. Oxford Press, New York. 1999.

Tsouna-Hadjis, E. et al. First stroke recovery process: the role of family social support. *Archives of Physical Medicine and Rehabilitation.* 2000;81(7): 881-7.

Wallace, RK. Physiological effects of transcendental meditation. *Science.* 1970 March;167(3926): 1751-1754.

For sales, editorial information, subsidiary rights information
or a catalog, please write or phone or e-mail
Brick Tower Press
1230 Park Avenue, 9a
New York, NY 10128, US
Sales: 1-800-68-BRICK
Tel: 212-427-7139
www.BrickTowerPress.com
email: bricktower@aol.com.

www.Ingram.com

CPSIA information can be obtained at www.ICGtesting.com
Printed in the USA
BVOW021800250312

286014BV00001B/29/P